# TECHNOLOGY AND NURSING

# Technology and Nursing

## Practice, Concepts and Issues

Edited by

Alan Barnard and Rozzano Locsin

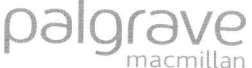

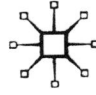

First published in 2007 by
PALGRAVE MACMILLAN
Houndmills, Basingstoke, Hampshire RG21 6XS and
175 Fifth Avenue, New York, N.Y. 10010
Companies and representatives throughout the world.

PALGRAVE MACMILLAN is the global academic imprint of the Palgrave Macmillan division of St. Martin's Press, LLC and of Palgrave Macmillan Ltd. Macmillan® is a registered trademark in the United States, United Kingdom and other countries. Palgrave is a registered trademark in the European Union and other countries.

ISBN-13: 978–1–4039–4649–2
ISBN-10: 1–4039–4649–3

This book is printed on paper suitable for recycling and made from fully managed and sustained forest sources. Logging, pulping and manufacturing processes are expected to conform to the environmental regulations of the country of origin.

A catalogue record for this book is available from the British Library.

10  9  8  7  6  5  4  3  2  1
16  15  14  13  12  11  10  09  08  07

Printed in China

*For my mother and father, Jeanine and Gordon Barnard,*
*who taught me the great value of perseverance and probity*

Alan Barnard

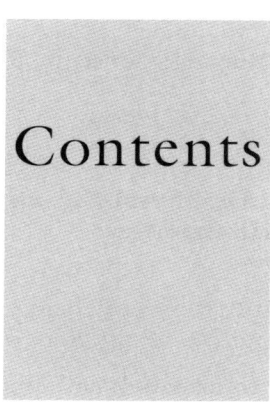

# Contents

# List of Figures

# List of Tables

# Acknowledgements

Every attempt has been made to trace and acknowledge copyright, but in some cases this may not have been possible. The publisher apologises for any accidental infringements and would welcome any information to redress this situation.

# Notes on Contributors

**Alan Barnard**, RN, BA, MA, PhD, Senior Lecturer, School of Nursing, Queensland University of Technology, Queensland, Australia.

**Susan Beidler**, RN, PhD, Assistant Professor of Nursing, Florida Atlantic University, Boca Raton, Florida.

**Aric S. Campling**, RN, MS, Clinical Information Systems Analyst, Children's Hospital, Boston.

**Susan Chase**, RN, EdD, Associate Professor of Nursing, Florida Atlantic University, Boca Raton, Florida.

**Moya Conrick**, RN, RM, DAppSc (NursEd), BN, MClEd, PhD Lecturer, Griffith University, Queensland, Australia.

**Kathryn B. Keller**, RN, PhD, Assistant Professor, Christine E. Lynn College of Nursing, Florida Atlantic University, Boca Raton, Florida.

**Rozzano Locsin**, RN, PhD, FAAN, Professor, Christine E. Lynn College of Nursing, Florida Atlantic University, Boca Raton, Florida.

**Jacqueline Lopez-Devine**, RN, PhD, Associate Professor of Nursing, Christine E. Lynn College of Nursing, Florida Atlantic University, Boca Raton, Florida.

**Paula Proctor**, RN, MSc, Reader in Nursing, School of Nursing, University of Sheffield, United Kingdom.

**Deborah Raines**, RNC, PhD, Professor, Christine E. Lynn College of Nursing, Florida Atlantic University, Boca Raton, Florida.

**Marilyn Ray,** RN, PhD, Professor, Christine E. Lynn College of Nursing, Florida Atlantic University, Boca Raton, Florida.

**Bob Ribbons,** RN, ICCert, BAppSc (Nur), MEd (Computing), Clinical Informatician, Manager of Clinical Informatics, Peninsula Health, Melbourne, Australia.

**Rose Sherman,** EdD, RN, CNAA, Director of the Nursing Leadership Institute, Christine E. Lynn College of Nursing at Florida Atlantic University, Boca Raton, Florida.

**Margarette Somerville,** RN, RSCN, HiTeC Coordinator, Xavier Children's Support Network, Australia.

**Tetsuya Tanioka**, RN, PhD, Associate Professor, Department of Community and Psychiatric Nursing, Faculty of Health Sciences, The University of Tokushima, Tokushima, Japan.

**Katherine Wang,** RN, PhD, Assistant Professor, School of Nursing, Yang-Ming University in Taipei, Taiwan.

**Carol Windsor,** RN, BA (Hons), Lecturer, School of Nursing, Queensland University of Technology, Queensland, Australia.

# Glossary of Terms

- **Division of labour:** Generally refers to the organisation of labour around prescribed tasks and roles for the purposes of increasing efficiency in productive output.

- **Holism:** Relates to ecology which looks at living and non-living things as wholes in the universe but also how wholes are embedded in larger wholes to arrive at the highest common bond of the universe and humanity.

- **Holonomy:** The study of the interrelationship between parts and whole where the properties of the parts (explicate order) can only be understood from the dynamics of the whole (implicate order).

- **Knowing persons:** A deliberate and intentional process of nursing in which persons are consciously acknowledged as whole, dynamic and unpredictable in the moment. This circuitous process is expressed as the nurse continuously assesses the person as whole and complete from one moment to the next moment.

- **Person:** A whole, dynamic and unpredictable human being who is complete in the moment (Boykin & Schoenhofer, 2001).

- **Sciences of Complexity:** Complexity sciences are scientific dynamical theories that illuminate the interconnectedness of all things in the universe. These illuminate dynamic interconnectedness, the ontology of holism and the notion of chaos – disorder and order where disorder and order of complex systems at the edge of chaos transform to either disintegrate or self-organise.

- **Technique:** The maximisation of efficiency and order in nursing, health care and society through the integration of human, organisational, political and economic systems.

- **Technology:** Artefacts, resources and their complex interrelationship with knowledge, skill, science, people, organisations, systems, culture, values and politics. Technology is advanced for purposes of survival, transmission of cultural values, development of societies, economic gain, political leadership, military power, maintenance of health, the giving and receiving of information and exploration.

- **Technological competency:** Technological competency is the practice of using health care technologies for the purpose of knowing persons in an efficient and appropriate manner.

- **Technology-dependent children:** The Office of Technology Assessment of the United States of America (OTA) defines a technology-dependent child as one who requires both a medical device to compensate for the loss of a vital body function and significant and sustained care in order to avert death or further disability.

- **Technological determinism:** Assumes technology is largely self-determining or an autonomous force that powerfully influences society without in turn being shaped by society.

- **Telecare:** The wider application of telematics to the whole healthcare environment, and involves (e.g.) management and nursing, as well as medical information transfer.

- **Telehealth:** Telehealth is the delivery of health-related services, enabled by the innovative use of technology, such as videoconferencing, without the need for travel.

- **Telematics:** The use of telecommunication in conjunction with informatics, (e.g.) the passing of information from one computer to another via a telephone line or other electronic link.

- **Telenursing:** The use of telecommunications for nursing care.

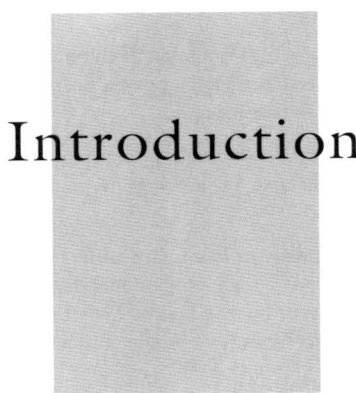

# Introduction

This book examines the way nursing relates to the development of technology in health care. It emphasises three things: the reasons to be excited yet cautious about technology, the challenges and advantages of technology for health care, and an insight into nursing care expressed by colleagues dedicated to inquiring into the influence of technology.

In keeping with the growth in examining technology, the emphasis of this book is on assisting clinical practice and looking at the emerging understanding of technology. Health care work requires skilled practitioners who are technically competent, and have the ability to foster healthier individuals and communities through adaptation, well-being and appropriate use of technology. The task of including advancing technology in nursing and health care is immensely important, yet it remains a challenge to all. Technology is present everywhere we practise and live, yet we are not always aware of it. It seems to be with us, yet not always at the forefront of our awareness. We use hundreds, if not thousands, of machines and equipment every day and we agree to follow policies and recommended procedures, yet amongst all these activities clinical practice and technology can remain commonplace. The technology of nursing, especially technology associated with basic or standard nurse intervention and body care, is concealed often from our reflection even though it is a part of us. In fact, it is not until technology is revealed for its lack of application or failure to respond to our needs that we notice it. In such cases, we might comment that 'the intravenous infusion pump will not work', 'my watch has stopped', 'the bed linen is wet' or 'this cup is leaking'. Technology is here with us, yet it seemingly has a life of its own that we occasionally notice and engage with it in a reflective way. The views expressed within this book seek to confront these experiences, highlight the great benefits of technology for health care and encourage you to engage in deeper critical reflection on its influence. Our aims are for you, the reader, to be introduced to some of the insights, experience and theories of practitioners and scholars in nursing. When it comes to technology, we want to impress on you the great need to consider further ways to enhance care and for you to consider perspectives on practice development and future advances for health care. The book is not meant to be exhaustive in its coverage but is meant to provide needed consideration of important health care developments. It is hoped that you will agree that ongoing examination of technology offers improved person- and community-focused care. Every contributor wants to impress upon you the great value of developing professional perspectives that are inspired by an awareness of technology within the broad context of health care and society and the new ways by which health care leaders might influence care in the future.

The book includes the voices of practising nurses, scholars and researchers from numerous countries and seeks to join together the thoughts of many in a discussion on technology. In each chapter readers are invited to engage in reflection and analysis on selected topics. The first two chapters of the book set the scene conceptually and convey insights drawn from theory to inform readers of important foundation knowledge. The focus is on technology as a social and professional phenomenon within the context of nursing and health care. The discussion presents frameworks for understanding technology and the relation between technology and competence. Complexity of experience and interpretation is highlighted by Alan Barnard as he examines *what is technology*, and both Rozanno Locsin and Alan Barnard consider technological competency as an expression of caring in nursing. Alan emphasises the importance of a broad description of technology, the central role that technology has always played in the development of clinical practice and how influential the characteristics of technology are upon our behaviour, thinking and care outcomes. Rozanno and Alan also explain that when integrating technology in health care and nursing practice three concepts need to be part of understanding, that is, wholeness of persons in the moment, knowing persons and technological competency as caring. It is noted that because technology is a part of practice it has become a measure of nursing achievement and part of our ongoing commitment to the needs of the health care sector. It is emphasised that we must consider the meaning of technology and our expression of caring since these are necessary for appropriate person-focused care. In the next chapter, Deborah Raines and Kathryn Keller note that technology is both a benefit and a burden. As a result of reflection on their clinical practice, they highlight the effect technology has upon the organisation of care, knowledge, change and skills. They note that technology pushes us to understand new concepts, to approach old problems in novel ways, to master the use of new devices and to learn to interpret results. They note increased accountability, respectability and greater autonomy within the restrictions of policy and protocol. Deborah and Kathryn stress that as has always been the case the challenge for the intensive care nurse, now and in the future, is to find a balance between the use of technologies and professional caring behaviours. Strategies such as family presence during resuscitation are suggested as appropriate practice examples and models for future care because they highlight the potential for humanised practice even in the midst of technology. The authors make points important to your practice as advanced technology becomes increasingly a part of both intensive care and a range of care contexts.

Following on from this chapter we move to a chapter by Susan Beidler and Susan Chase who highlight that maintaining the ethical integrity of interactions between patients and nurses is increasingly a challenge as new modes of communication and health information systems become commonplace. With the development of computers, Internet and distance technology, creative and unique ways of delivering health information and health care services are emerging that challenge traditional behaviours, skills and knowledge. The chapter addresses issues such as protection of patient information, duty to provide care, patient abandonment, risks and benefits of telehealth nursing and identification of reputable health-related Internet sites. Strategies and suggestions for upholding the legal and ethical traditions of nursing while interfacing with latest technology-assisted patient–nurse interactions are included to assist the reader. Exemplars included in the chapter illustrate choices and decisions that influence patient care outcomes and demonstrate integration of technology in health care. The chapter concludes by highlighting future priority areas and recommendations for emerging health policy.

Kathryn Wang, Alan Barnard and Margarette Somerville are also concerned about changing contexts of care. In their chapter they highlight the importance of persons in care and how community care, particularly for children, is greatly affected by the use of advanced medical equipment in unfamiliar environments such as the home. Kathryn, Alan and Margarette explain that technology-dependent children when discharged home have a direct impact on the lives of all individuals in the home. Through qualitative research the authors describe how psychological and social support for one group of children and their families needed to be a focus for health care professionals. Support of family and child is shown to aid family stability, care provision and the promotion of quality of life for a child, each person caring for a child, and their family. The chapter shows how technology is much more than medical supplies, equipment and machinery, and is linked directly to alteration of personal and social values as well as alteration of human relations.

As we consider care provision, communication and altered physical boundaries of health care delivery, we take a further step in the next chapter into new environments to consider human–humanoid communication and partnerships. Aric Campling, Tetsuya Tanioka and Rozanno Locsin outline emerging relationships between robots (anthropomorphic machines), technological competence and changes in the scope and provision of health care. Their discussion stresses the implications for nursing and health care of *machines* with human-like characteristics and of *human beings* with technological parts such as pacemakers and artificial limbs. The chapter introduces the reader to emerging social and professional issues in relation to implications of current developments for nursing and interdisciplinary teams and the future role of robots in clinical practice and health care.

Following on from Aric, Tetsuya and Rozanno, Paula Proctor explores the uses of telematics in the United Kingdom health care system. Paula highlights the application of tele-triage through the use of a nurse-led national call centre, telecare through the use of support infrastructure for carers in their own home, tele-patient education/support through mobile (cell) technology and tele-education through the delivery of workshops across two continents. The chapter begins with a historical overview of the use of computers to support health care in the United Kingdom. Paula highlights that nursing can demonstrate a lead role in an ever increasing number of 'tele-' developments and notes both great success and questionable effectiveness. It is observed that as we progress further into the twenty-first century it is likely that more use will be made of telehealth but significant work is needed by nurses to maximise the potential benefits of this type of technology for health care gains.

In the next chapter we move from the community to the hospital context. Jacqueline Lopez-Devine and Rose Sherman outline changes associated with the integration of a computer-based patient care system into a large hospital in United States of America. Successful adoption is highlighted, but they stress that despite the urgency of integrating information technology with health care delivery and management, when compared to progress made in other industries, health care has been slow to adopt computerised technology for patient care systems. Jacqueline and Rose argue that we nurses are now more technologically confident with respect to modern electronic and computerised equipment than nurses of the past. Advancements in technology, improvements in computer hardware and the use of integrated information systems can facilitate development within health professions. We learn of the implications of the Information System Life Cycle, the lessons learned from a case study looking at computer integration in clinical practice, the potential value of applying Everett Roger's Adoption of Innovation Theory as a framework for nursing and health care and overview nursing research and issues related to protection of patient information, duty to provide care, the challenges and benefits of telehealth nursing and the identification of reputable health-related Internet sites.

In the next chapter Moya Conrick and Bob Ribbons explain the relation between information technology and the creation, storage, exchange and use of data, information and knowledge. Computers and information technology are often claimed to support improvements to the management of health information and our delivery of patient care. Moya and Bob show, however, that information systems are highly political and are central to the maintenance of huge volumes of people and information in increasingly high acuity health care environments, despite limited evidence and support for their effectiveness in some areas of health care delivery. High volume and complexity of health care data places increasing pressure on nurses. We require advanced communication and political skills grounded in human-centred models that stress acquisition, processing, storage and dissemination of information for quality care that is more than just information retrieval.

In the final three chapters we shift our attention to broader consideration of clinical practice in the light of labour force development and knowledge development for nursing. Carol Windsor begins by stressing the need for greater recognition of nursing endeavour as work and stresses that technologies and technological change in nursing cannot be treated separately from an understanding of nursing work as socially defined, shaped and organized. Carol highlights the need to identify nursing work as *work*, and examines the effects of broader institutional and organisational change on nursing practice using an approach derived from political economy. The limitations of contemporary approaches in considering technological development in nursing are highlighted especially for their weakness in explaining the role of technology in nursing and changing division of nursing labour as the principle drivers of change.

In the next chapter Alan Barnard argues that future directions in health care must be informed by further research and scholarship. Alan emphasises that specific analysis of technology is required that relies less on claims of dehumanisation, determinism and uncritical celebration of technological change, and more on considered analysis of specific relations between technology, nursing care, persons and health care practices. He shows how evidence and considered argument is increasingly needed in health care; why sustainable and effective health initiatives are important and supports a re-invigoration of cultural, spiritual, moral and social values. Finally, Marilyn Ray asks us also to consider technology as a relational phenomenon. Marilyn explains that technology is advancing for purposes of survival, transmission of cultural values, development of societies, economic gain, political leadership, military power, maintenance of health and the giving and receiving of information and exploration. Amongst all these purposes and change Marilyn notes is the experience of technology in nursing practice and its relation to the meaning of embodiment. The author asks us to consider whether there is a key to grasping the relations between technology and caring in nursing practice. Marilyn searches for possible answers in the precepts of the sciences of complexity, the meaning of the personal and the professional in nursing, technology as a relational phenomenon, the experience of 'presence-at-hand' and presencing and finally technological caring as co-creative emergence portraying both the onto-theological and the ethics of trust (faith, hope and love). Marilyn advances the view that we must continue to seek to address questions of the interrelationship between technology and caring and stresses that technological caring is the gift of one's being to the other and the interpenetration of each person in each other's lives.

The perspectives outlined in this book are more than an account of current practice. They express a concern for the questions *what sort of world should we nurses be co-constructing?* and amongst all the change, *do we engage with, and think about, technology in ways that best inform our practice and health care?* Limited evidence has been documented in nursing history and contemporary care that expresses an appreciation for the direct impact of technology on our individual and collective practice. The authors argue that technology is significant. This realisation brings with it growing practice, intellectual, professional, ethical, economic and political responsibilities. The identification of technology as a major phenomenon requiring critical examination at this time is an endorsement of the necessity for us to express long overdue perspectives on technology that are linked to our values, actions and goals. This book emphasises consideration of practical application of technology across a range of health care areas and is one of the first books to highlight technology in nursing. We hope our readers are inspired by the contents of this book to engage in thinking about and using technology in ways that are best for every person and context. We focus deliberately on the experience and context of individuals, community and society, and are guided by a desire for compassionate and appropriate intervention and care.

ALAN BARNARD AND ROZANNO LOCSIN

# Advancing the Meaning of Nursing and Technology

## Alan Barnard

### LEARNING OBJECTIVES

When you have read this chapter, you will be able to:

- Discuss the meaning of nursing technology for nursing and health care
- Explain issues and concepts significant to the experience of technology
- Identify the importance of technology for clinical practice
- Discuss technology in relation to professional development and the organisation of health care

### KEY WORDS

- care
- clinical practice
- knowledge
- nursing
- skills
- technique
- technology
- theory

## 1.1 Breaching uncertainty

Technology plays an important part in nursing, society and health care. Although we use it in our everyday practice we are not always aware of technology unless there are malfunctions (e.g. an infusion pump continues to alarm despite your efforts to troubleshoot its function). Technology is important to our personal and professional lives but rarely does its presence lead us to ask ourselves, *what is technology* and *what meaning does it have for me, my colleagues and the people for whom I care*? This unseen(ness) and lack of examination makes sense because we are intensely involved with getting on with what we do as nurses, but it does reflect a commonplace lack of engagement with thinking about the implication and future of technology. Our professional roles and responsibilities encourage us to get on with our work. It is on occasions when we might lack time to be able to provide personal care because of technological demands, or at times when we have to take critical decisions that will affect a persons' health, that we experience greater awareness and clarity about the enormity of our roles and our relation with technology.

Reflection on technology is a specific focus of inquiry important for understanding and developing health care practice and services (Locsin, 2001; McConnell, 1995; Pellegrino & Thomasma, 1981; Reiser, 1978; Sandelowski, 2000; Starr, 1982). This chapter focuses on technology as a social and professional phenomenon and presents a way of explaining it within the context of nursing. It emphasises the importance of developing a good understanding of technology and the limitations of commonplace beliefs, and highlights what is necessary for critical interpretation and reflection.

### Technology and science

In many science-based disciplines technology has been defined as an applied science. Science is characterised as *knowing what* and technology as *knowing how*. Recent thinking about technology demonstrates that technology and science are two discrete bodies of knowledge (Cotgrove, 1982; Ihde, 1993; Mitcham, 1994; Purcell, 1994; Wajcman, 1991). The belief that science discovers and technology applies no longer survives serious scrutiny (Ellul, 1964; Ihde, 1993; Mumford, 1934). Many technological advances have originated from minimal understanding of science and some have proceeded far beyond scientific knowledge and rationale. The development of the first aircraft and steam engine are two commonly cited historical advancements in technology that evolved separate to scientific explanation (Brinkman, 1971; Mumford, 1934; Purcell, 1994). Within nursing an example has been the creation of aseptic procedures during the Crimean war that significantly reduced death rates. The practice advancements initiated by Florence Nightingale were made without any understanding of bacteria.

Whilst science provides technology with the knowledge and means for growth, it has not been essential for technological development from either a historical or a pre-conditional perspective. Both can claim to be two separate yet related bodies of knowledge, and in recent years science and technology are aligned increasingly and advances could easily be referred to as 'techno-science' (Ferre, 1995; Ihde, 1993; Purcell, 1994).

Technology is required to fit with the economic, human and material purposes of health care and nursing. It is valued sometimes as a status symbol because of its link(s) with science and is associated with specialist expertise. There are clear patterns of life style, practice and cultural activity that identify technology as influential upon our lives.

## 1.2 Technology and nursing history

Before the twentieth century, nursing was essentially a craft practised mostly by women who gained experience through religious and secular orders or through family. Knowledge and skill developed by trial and error and were passed down through generations. Nursing practice relied upon rule of thumb, experience and faith. Specific practices were linked sometimes to isolated groups, individuals and geographic areas and included magical and aesthetic components that fitted with moral and cultural life. Nursing was provided by trusted individuals who provided care based less on scientific knowledge than on a personal and intuitive understanding, developed and refined through practice (Barnard & Cushing, 2001; Reverby, 1987).

Before the industrial revolution technology was slow to develop. Skills relied as much on technology as the know-how of a craft-person's expert eye. The slow development meant that technical advance rarely threatened social equilibrium and was assimilated into society and practice (Ellul, 1964; Mumford, 1934). The rapid growth of scientific and technical knowledge since the eighteenth century has generated enormous changes for nursing, health care and society. Technology and science have developed at a rate which is affecting every facet of our awareness and experience. The rapid growth of both science and technology present us with many challenges, particularly those associated with workplace and employment, pace of life, access to information, extended life span in affluent countries, increasing poverty and pollution, and adoration of technological change.

Like society, we nurses both welcome and encourage technological development. Belief in the benefits of technology has not, however, encouraged us to do much more than apply technology(ies) in care provision. We have not spent much time developing a historical awareness of the influence of technology upon nursing or understanding its significance (Harding, 1980; Reverby, 1987; Sandelowski, 1988). Historical texts, nursing literature and manuals of nursing practice fail to comment on the social and professional impact of technological change. Like many professional groups, we have ignored the social outcomes of technological development, and analysis has been limited to histories of technological advances in medicine. In addition, the importance of moral or ethical changes associated with technology, human experience of technology and analysis of the impact of technology upon society and groups has not been realised. Nursing history texts of the twentieth century which purported to analyse trends in nursing were inadequate in their reflection and analysis of technology. For example, we have specific knowledge of the experience of people who have health care technology as part of their treatment; we are involved intimately in decision making about care provision using technology; we are influential upon care outcomes; we have a role to play as leaders in the use and application of health care technology; we work in all the various parts of the health care system and are positioned to take a stronger role in thinking about, and responding to, complex health care issues and trends; we have a unique human focus in health care that can contribute a great deal to better care planning and policy.

Inadequate insight into the experience of technology continues to restrict the development of nursing as a discipline (Harding, 1980; Sandelowski, 2000). When we begin to properly see technology as influential in the organisation of human labour and fundamental to moral, practical and political goals we will find that there are many gains for us. A better understanding of technology is needed because current views contribute to 'ineffective and destructive interactions with nature and also support privileged access to the social benefits of technological change' (Harding, 1980, p. 56).

## 1.3 Expressing the meaning of nursing and technology

We make use of an enormous range of technology. In fact we practise in the midst of technology; nursing is significantly shaped by it and we act upon it as a phenomenon. A significant amount of technology is created by nurses, as evidenced by Sandelowski (2000) who demonstrated that American nurses in the modern era have had roles in inventing, designing and applying technology but which have most often been *un*recorded. It has only been in the past thirty years that nurses have begun to seriously examine technology. The relations between technology and nursing have been considered in theory and historical analysis, but more work is needed in the area (Barnard, 2001; Fairman & Lynaugh, 1998; Harding, 1980; Reverby, 1987; Sandelowski, 2000).

Explanation of technology in nursing has been problematic and many nurses reduce technology to a discrete thing or object (i.e. they essentialise technology – which means that they reduce understanding of technology to a single *entity* or *essence*). For example, a colleague might claim that technology is all the modern machinery used in the ward.

In addition, literature can assume that there is common understanding and, if it is defined, technology is described most commonly as practical tools, machinery and equipment (Hawthorne & Yurkovich 1995; Henderson, 1985; McClure, 1991; McConnell, 1990; Wichowski, 1994). For example, McClure (1991, p. 144) stated that technology is '... any means of delivering care using objects that are not a part of the patients own body. This means that it includes not only the vast array of machinery we have come to take for granted, but also the pharmaceuticals that are prescribed and administered'.

Technology has tended to be described in terms of socially stereotypical terms such as impressive machinery, industrial objects and scientific advances such as X-ray machinery or a cardiograph. Commonplace technology important to our practice such as enema cans, trolleys, beds, needles and uniforms have tended to remain hidden even though they reflect more closely the technology of the daily practice of nurses. This tendency has restricted a full understanding of technology and nursing in preference for a commonplace societal interpretation of the phenomenon. For example, societal explanation of technology has tended to trivialise technology(ies) associated with gendered activities such as childcare or cooking in order to stereotype women (who are commonly associated with these roles) as technologically incapable and ignorant (Wajcman, 1991).

There is limited research published that focuses on explanation of technology and the way(s) technology is integrated into clinical practice. Therefore, limited evidence exists to advance or refute various commonplace claims about the effectiveness of technology for nursing (e.g. technology is claimed to save us time and reduce the cost of care). Research is needed on the relations between technology and clinical practice; theoretical models; ongoing skills and knowledge advancement; and issues associated with power, gender, human experience and practice development (Barnard, 2001, 2002; Carnevali, 1985; Harding, 1980; Pelletier, 1989; Sandelowski, 1997, 2000; Walters, 1994; Zwolski, 1989). Nursing literature emphasises embellishment of scientific development, and there is an excessive amount of anecdotal opinion that lacks supporting evidence or theoretical foundation. Perspectives emphasise both technological determinism and technology as a neutral phenomenon.

## Technological determinism

Determinism is an extreme perspective that argues that personal responsibility and individual will/volition/agency are illusions because all actions and events are determined by other causal phenomena such as technology. Technological determinism argues that all human discovery and development has arisen from, and is subject to, technological change. If embraced, the belief (doctrine) can dominate our thinking about, for example, groups such as nursing, the development of civilizations and society (Bimber, 1994; Ellul, 1980; Feenberg, 1999; Ferre, 1995; Greaves & Wilmot, 2001; Winner, 1977). The belief is revealed in statements such as 'technology changes the way we nurse' or 'nurses must be responsive to the demands of technology'. It is a way of thinking that is found in not only fearful (dystopian) discussion about technology (i.e. worried about the effects of technology) (Calne, 1994; Donley, 1991), but also in overly embracing (utopian) discussion about technology (i.e. technology is responsible for creating perfect social and professional harmony) (Salmon, 1977; Simpson, 2003). McClure (1991, p. 144) expressed the enthusiasm shared by many when she noted that '... the steady and pervasive increase in technology advancement in health care during the twentieth century has been a source of excitement and constant pride to all of us in the field'.

A significant characteristic of the standpoint expressed by many nurses (McClure, 1991; Reed-Ash, 1983; Simpson & Brown, 1990) is thinking of technological progress as linear. Linear progress means that technology advances arithmetically (constantly and predictably) through an addition of constant differences (e.g. 0, 5, 10, 15, 20, etc.) to an ever greater and higher level. We are thus believed to be progressing ever upwards to greater achievement and success. The arguments supporting linear progress are fallacious yet they dominate nursing thought (Barnard, 1999; Herdman, 2001).

What is demanded from us is a balanced view. Technological development can be likened to the arts. Its history is noteworthy in terms of its periods of achievement, failure, advance and respite. There are contrasting periods of discovery, invention and failure. Progress relies generally on our collective knowledge and skills that randomly accumulate and come together to advance and retard technology and science (Ellul, 1964; Koestler, 1964; Mitcham, 1994; Mumford, 1934; Winner, 1977).

Clinical environments sometimes struggle to provide emotional support for patients and families. There is sometimes a marginalization of chronic illness, increasing demand for efficiency and effectiveness, and an over-reliance on machinery and equipment. These effects combined with increasing legal liability associated with health care and the maintenance of machinery, and so forth, produce an emphasis on function, policy, safety, protocol and specialization. However, to characterise nurses as little more than technicians in an inhuman world (Braun et al., 1984; Calne, 1994; Cooper, 1993, 1994; Donley, 1991; Henderson, 1985; Kelly, 2004; Laing, 1982; Sandelowski, 1988; West, 2003; Wilkin & Slevin, 2004) where people are secondary to the needs of institutions and the technology that controls them is incorrect and destructive.

Similar determinist opinion can be found also from a utopian perspective. Technological and scientific knowledge does enable us to be more responsible in health care but it does not make us professionals, as some authors have claimed (McClure, 1991; Simpson, 2002; Simpson & Brown, 1990). For example, Simpson and Brown (1985, p. 62) implore us to embrace technology as an influential force in determining the development of nursing: 'Technology advances are being made at an astounding rate and will have a profound impact upon nursing practice. The profession of nursing must be prepared to take advantage of this technology and use it to determine its own destiny'.

What is best stated about the influence of technology is that technological advancements can be linked to changes in health care and have enabled us to develop new expertise and roles. Technology is associated with an increased need for education and leadership by nurses and our roles are influenced by many of the associated characteristics of technology, which include a drive for efficiency, protocols, equipment change, skills alteration and electronic sophistication. The way we respond to these characteristics will, in large part, reflect our ability to understand technology and specific ways to integrate it appropriately into our goals and practices.

## The neutral perspective

All changes come with both a benefit and a cost. Evidence demonstrates that technology does influence our practice, values and environment often without due recognition of the importance of the transformation (Barnard, 1997; Feenberg, 1999; Reiser, 1986; Sandelowski, 2000). For example, in a study by Wilkin and Slevin (2004) it was found that although intensive-care nurses do identify the gaining of knowledge and skills as essential for technological competence the participants highlighted that psychological care of patients can sometimes be overshadowed by technology. It was noted that technology assists to meet physical needs but simultaneously reduces other dimensions of care and experience. Despite these types of experiences many of us continue to believe that technology has limited unplanned effect upon our action and views. That is, that technology has no ability to determine our behaviour, values or clinical practice. This belief in the neutral impact of technology is expressed in common statements such as 'machines do not make decisions they only solve problems', 'humans discover problems and mechanise efficient resolutions' or 'technology intervenes after thinking has been finished in order to serve us'. Apparently, 'good nurses' are well organised and are never influenced by technology in their care (Ashworth, 1987; Carnevali, 1985; Gordon, 1992; Henderson, 1985; Johnson, 2000; McClure, 1991; Orem, 1991; Salmon, 1969; Simpson, 2003). These views encourage us to believe that technology is just an agent of use that is independent of human action and choice. Problems in practice reflect inadequacy in the way machinery and equipment are used by you or your team (i.e. good workers never blame their tools). Issues related to politics, ethics, morals and individual action are considered separate to technology. According to Cotgrove (1982) the belief in the neutral effect of technology is a dominant sociological paradigm that emphasises domination and mastery. It strengthens the argument that humans have the right and the ability to manipulate nature for their own desired ends and purposes. It demands a faith in technology, science and scientific method, and directs us to view technology uncritically as the champion of health care services and professional development. Carnevali (1985) is typical of nurses who espouse a faith in the belief: '... for the sake of both the client and clinician it would seem sound to consider technology a basic, neutral concept' (p. 12).

However, the technology of many nursing environments alters habits, intentions, judgements, thoughts, needs, plans and personal preferences. For example, alarms are notorious for the way they unreservedly call our attention during even the most important or intense periods of the day. It is not unusual to have to leave doing something or speaking with someone to have to attend to an alarm originating from a devise or monitor. That is what alarms are designed to do! They are supposed to alter your attention and activity in order to have you answer 'the call'.

We are required to use a lot of machines, equipment and tools and to fulfil the requirements of an increasing array of protocols, competencies and organisational policy. Can we truly claim that we are masters when the complexity of technology is examined in its entirety? Belief in a neutral influence of technology robs us of opportunity. Technology is complex and our practice environment has been long modified before any claim of independence, control or choice. For example, consider the increasing number of protocols, practice directives and standardised care plans that exist in many hospital environments. They seek to direct the way you should practise. Whilst many are an advantage, especially if you are inexperienced, they do come at a cost. You no longer need to necessarily plan or investigate alternative approaches since you are directed already to behave in a certain way.

A neutral argument leads us to overlook technology as a powerful political influence and an important site of inter-disciplinary tension. Neutrality emphasises the immediateness of technical action without fostering our need or desire to adequately reflect on the breadth of technological development and its influence on nursing and health care.

## 1.4  The meaning of technology for nursing

How should we interpret technology given all the competing interests and emerging implications? Contrary to popular belief technology is not simple to explain. To address the challenge, it is argued that we need to not define technology but identify its characteristics as a way of explanation. That is, we need to understand the characteristics of technology rather than lay claim to a definitive account because technology cannot be reduced to a single thing or essence. That being said, however, I recognise it is necessary to communicate a meaning of technology for the purposes of this chapter and book. Clearly, technology influences our lives, and its obvious effect can be witnessed in our action, skills and knowledge. Technology represents our accumulation of knowledge over centuries arising from intelligent discovery and is influenced by design, gender, science, social relations, culture, values and politics (Dunphy, 1985; Ellul, 1964; Feenberg, 1999, 2003; Marck, 2000; Mitcham, 1989, 1994; Wajcman, 1991).

A way to explain each characteristic of technology is to portray them diagrammatically as three concentric circles (Figure 1.1). Concentric circles are useful because they highlight our 'tools of trade' at the centre of our experience but emphasise that technology is much more. Each concentric circle represents characteristics of technology, and together the circles express what *is* technology (Barnard, 1998).

### Artefact and resources of nursing

The smallest concentric central circle entitled 'artefact and resources' is technology at its most obvious. It denotes tools, equipment, machinery and other ways technology appears in the form of resources, electronic devices, gadgets, computers, automata, information and the various means at our disposal for the daily enactment of nursing (e.g. sphygmomanometers, infusion pumps, beds, electricity, pharmaceuticals, gas, trolleys, digital screens, urinals, trays, syringes, bedpan sluice, dressing packs, automata and uniforms).

An artefact can include antibiotics, needles, industrial materials; communications technology and pharmaceutics. The *things themselves* are the focal or central point of attention and they express the coming together of our thought, ideas,

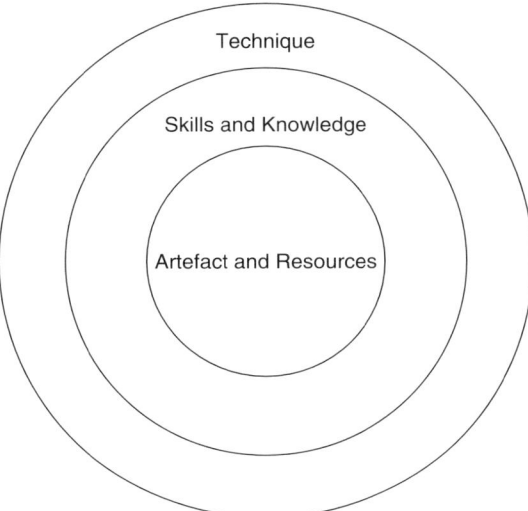

**Figure 1.1**   Characteristics of technology.

invention and activity. Often artefact and resources are the background (i.e. frame of reference) from which many other experiences and understandings emerge (Barnard & Gerber, 1999).

## Knowledge and skills

The second or middle concentric circle portrays technology as knowledge and skills. Meaning is conveyed to technology as a result of our experience and associated knowledge and skills that determine the way we use, repair and design it. At this level we make valued judgements about technology and form beliefs about its use and application. At this level issues of technological competence, the necessity for ongoing education and personal development, the changing nature of nursing knowledge and skills and the relations between practice and caring are most apparent. It is at this level that we think about how we practice, what knowledge we require, how specialist areas differ and what are the goals of nursing in rapidly changing and developing environments.

An artefact such as a bedpan is as much technology as the knowledge and skills necessary for its use. For example, without necessary knowledge and skills to inform a nurse about the use of an intravenous infusion pump it is little more to the nurse than plastic, metal and electricity. If the nurse attempts to use the technology without requisite knowledge and skills the outcomes of care provision are likely to be dangerous and unprofessional. There will be constriction to the nurse's clinical judgment(s) that will affect curative and caring practice(s). Knowledge and skills are essential for the achievement of acceptable practice standards, ethical decisions, professional accountability, personal responsibility and practice advancement. Knowledge and skills are therefore fundamentally linked with technology as an artefact and resource.

Technology is about changing skills and knowledge. To put it simply, your ability to use, for example, a bedpan or an intravenous infusion pump is dependent on educational and professional preparation for the role and responsibility. The use of technology in clinical practice relates specifically to a readiness and ability to express technological competency necessary for the advancement of appropriate care.

## Technique

The third and most inclusive concentric circle on the outer edge of Figure 1.1 refers to the concept of *technique*. It is at this level that our characteristics of technology arrive at political, economic and human concerns that inform, advance or impinge upon our beliefs and practice(s). Technique is not a thing, but is a way of thinking. Technique is a word that refers to the ways artefacts, resources, knowledge and skills are organised in an effort to reach maximum efficiency in action and create rational and logical order in our world. Technique reduces the means of production, whether they be machines, tools, skills, policy, knowledge or nurses, to that which is most technological (i.e. efficient and ordered) so as to join their function together on a daily and ongoing basis. Technique seeks to govern tools, equipment, resources, design, science, social alliance(s), organisations, economics, culture, values and politics in an effort to create predictable order and efficient practice.

Activity that was once tentative, unconscious and spontaneous is transformed to the realm of clear, voluntary and rational concepts and actions. For example, a caring moment with a person (e.g. patient) that is often motivated and informed by nothing more or less than compassion and concern for another is not a technology, whereas the premeditated use of efficient communication strategies for the fulfilment of predefined goals has all the hallmarks of a technology. Examples of this type of technology (technique) are economic rationalism, efficiency drives, communication strategies, time and motion studies, benchmarking, patient-dependency models, systems theory, diagnostic related groups and standardised nursing care plans.

The way in which our practice is organised *for*, as well as *by* machinery and tools, and so forth, is as much technology. There is nothing secondary about the ways technique organises the world around us (Ellul, 1964; Feenberg, 1999; Mitcham, 1994; Winner, 1977). The inclusion of artefacts and resources in nursing care introduces patterns of activity and knowledge that by their very nature alter practice and care. Interestingly, it must be noted that we are generally not exceptionally bothered by many of these changes because society prepares us for the experience. We expect activities to be devised in accordance with technique. We each gain the reassurance of being part of a health care system that is exemplified by the predictable nature of its control and efficiency. But when expectations or participation is not appropriate, particularly if human-centred care is not valued or able to be expressed, then there can be a feeling that health care practices are excessively standardised (Barnard, 2001, 2002; Peacock & Nolan, 2000). Technique is the creation of social and professional systems necessary for technology to progress. Systems are not simply theoretical;

they are sociological. Technique clarifies, arranges, reduces, rationalises and makes care efficient.

For example, Reiser (1978, p. 228) noted that health care practices and medical intervention are associated increasingly with the two qualities of reproducibility and standardisation. Reproducibility of practice treatment leads to accuracy and permanency, and standardisation enhances uniformity of interpretation and measurement. These developments decrease controversy, remove subjectivity and establish measures to make clinical practice reliable. Through technique a transformation is occurring in which many aspects of practice, even those that were once instinctive, reflexive, natural and particular to individuals and cultures, are being transformed into rational method and instruction.

Whilst technique has advantages, it creates environments that are typical for their standardisation, predictability, rigidity, sameness and universality. It may be necessary to encourage this in, for example, an emergency department, but if a flexible clinical care environment is appropriate the first move towards self-determination and some relaxation of technique is identification of the problem. Central to meaningful engagement with people and the establishment of a technological competence is recognition that we are not often free to go about all our activities making independent decisions and choices. We do so within guidelines, systems and policy.

Second, we need, where appropriate, to reject the idea that we must control every human activity. We each need to ask ourselves regularly and seriously what gives meaning in lives, nursing and the persons for whom we care. Once understood, we need to foster a certain detachment to the importance of technique and renewed respect for human experience. We must be willing at every stage to be certain of the reasons why we do things, the necessity and appropriateness of choices that are made, the suitability of care provided and the necessity to seek out something different where necessary.

Third, there is need for a concerted effort to reflect upon our nursing care and the importance of genuinely responding not only to the needs of institutions, but also to the needs and requirements of individuals and families. We need to engage in discussion about the impact of technique and seek to influence where possible organisations and decision makers.

## Technology and nursing

The approach for understanding technology outlined in this chapter directs us towards a deeper and more holistic interpretation. Available research demonstrates clearly that nurse education, research and practice must address issues related to not only the use of artefacts and resources, but also the way technology influences practice environments, the efforts of nurses to control practice, patient assessment and the reasonableness of seeking appropriate application of technology (Locsin, 2001; Sandelowski, 2000; Walters, 1994). Commonplace assumptions about technology are simplistic and do not assist us. This chapter has emphasised interpretation that stresses critical understanding of the development of nursing within the context of technologically complex health care systems and society (Barnard, 1997, 1999; Harding, 1980; Sandelowski, 1988, 1997).

The interpretation is important for the next stage of our development as practitioners and leaders in health care.

## 1.5 Final reflection

This chapter has presented a framework for understanding that illustrates the complexity of experience and interpretation. You have been asked to respond to the question *what is technology?* In beginning to answer the question from a nursing perspective, I have highlighted the relationship between characteristics of technology. It has been noted that technology has become a measure of nursing success and continues to be a modern response to the needs and goals of patients, nurses and society.

The relations between technology, nursing practice and patient-care outcomes are complex and significant. Responsible and advanced decision making informed by an appreciation for the characteristics of technology increases the possibility for excellence in care. We must now continue our commitment to interpreting technology. Accounts of the way in which technology is experienced and utilised by engineers, designers, testers and institutional workers are required (Pinch, 1991). The common thing is to be critical of scholarship that aims to analyse technology but to do nothing about the lack of research and serious reflection (Ellul, 1963; Pinch, 1991; Sklair, 1971). With continued commitment to understanding technology we will be better prepared to positively influence the quality of health care.

**LEARNING ACTIVITIES**

1. In a small group, discuss your shared experiences of technology that draw on a number of its characteristics. List strategies to foster appropriate integration of technology in clinical practice.

2. Debate the impact of technology on nurses. For example, how do our impressions about technology affect nursing practice? Why?

3. In small groups report on the implications of organisational policy and protocols for nursing care. List ways to meet the needs of health care organisations whilst maximising person-focused and appropriate care.

## References

Ashworth, P. (1987). Technology and machines – bad masters but good servants. *Intensive Care Nursing, 3*, 1–2.

Barnard, A. (1997). A critical review of the belief the technology is a neutral object and nurses are its master. *Journal of Advanced Nursing, 26*, 126–131.

Barnard, A. (1998). Understanding technology in contemporary surgical nursing: a phenomenographic examination. PhD Thesis. Faculty of Professional and Health Studies. The University of New England, Armidale, Australia.

Barnard, A. (1999). Nursing and the primacy of technological progress. *International Journal of Nursing Studies, 36,* 435–442.

Barnard, A. (2001). On the relationship between technique and dehumanization. In R. Locsin (ed.), *Advancing Technology, Caring and Nursing.* Westport, CT: Auburn House, pp. 96–105.

Barnard, A. (2002). Philosophy of technology and nursing. *Nursing Philosophy, 3,* 15–26.

Barnard, A. & Cushing, A. (2001). Technology and historical inquiry in nursing. In R. Locsin (ed.), *Advancing Technology, Caring and Nursing.* Westport, CT: Auburn House, pp. 12–21.

Barnard, A. & Gerber, R. (1999). Understanding technology in contemporary surgical nursing: a phenomenographic examination. *Nursing Inquiry, 6,* 157–170.

Bimber, B. (1994). Three faces of technological determinism. In M. R. Smith & L. Marx (ed.), *Does Technology Drive History?* Cambridge: The MIT Press, pp. 79–100.

Braun, J. L., Baines, S. L., Olson, N. G., Scruby, L. S., Manteuffel, C. A., & Cretilli, P. K. (1984). The future of nursing: Combining humanistic and technological values. *Health Values: Achieving High Level Wellness, 8*(3), 12–15.

Brinkman, D. (1971). Technology as philosophic problem. *Philosophy Today, 15*(2), 122–128.

Calne, S. (1994). Dehumanisation in intensive care. *Nursing Times, 90,* 31–33.

Carnevali, D. L. (1985). Nursing perspectives in health care technology. *Nursing Administration Quarterly, 9,* 10–18.

Cooper, M. C. (1993). The intersection of technology and care in the ICU. *Advances in Nursing Science, 15*(3), 23–32.

Cooper, M. C. (1994). Care: antidote for nurses' love–hate relationship with technology. *American Journal of Critical Care, 3,* 402–403.

Cotgrove, S. (1982). *Catastrophe or Cornucopia: The Environment, Politics and the Future.* New York: John Wiley.

Donley, R. (1991). Spiritual dimensions of health care: nursing mission. *Nursing & Health Care, 12,* 178–183.

Dunphy, D. C. (1985). Technological change and its impact on industrial democracy. *Work and People, 11*(2), 17–20.

Ellul, J. (1963). The technological order. In C. F. Stover (ed.), *The Technological Order.* Detroit, MI: Wayne State University Press.

Ellul, J. (1964). *The Technological Society.* New York: Alfred A Knopf.

Ellul, J. (1980). *The Technological System.* New York: Continuum.

Fairman, J. & Lynaugh, J. (1998). *Critical Care Nursing: A History.* Philadelphia, PA: The University of Pennsylvania Press.

Feenberg, A. (1999). *Questioning Technology.* New York: Routledge.

Feenberg, A. (2003). Modernity theory and technology studies: reflections on bridging the gap. In T. J. Misa, P. Brey, & A. Feenberg (eds), *Modernity and Technology.* MIT Press: Massachusetts, pp. 73–104.

Ferre, F. (1995). *Philosophy of Technology.* London: The University of Georgia Press.

Gordon, S. (1992). The importance of being nurses. *Technology Review, 95*(7), 42–51.

Greaves, J. P. & Wilmot, S. (2001). Demand pull or technology push: which is influencing change in nursing care and information practice? In R. Locsin (ed.), *Advancing Technology, Nursing and Caring.* Westport, CT: Auburn House, pp. 161–169.

Harding, S. (1980). Value laden technologies and the politics of nursing. In S. F. Spicker & S. Gadow (eds), *Nursing: Images and Ideals.* New York: Springer, pp. 49–75.

Hawthorne, D. L. & Yurkovich, N. J. (1995). Science, technology, caring and the professions: Are they compatible? *Journal of Advanced Nursing, 21,* 1087–1091.

Henderson, V. (1985). The essence of nursing in high technology. *Nursing Administration Quarterly, 9*(4), 1–9.

Herdman, E. (2001). The illusion of progress in nursing. *Nursing Philosophy, 2,* 4–13.

Ihde, D. (1993). *Philosophy of Technology: An Introduction.* Indiana, IN: Indiana University Press.

Johnson, P. (2000). Considering technology: Living and working in a technological society. *Journal of Midwifery & Women's Health, 45*(1), 79–80.

Kelly, J. (2004). Accountability and recent developments in nursing. *Dimensions of Critical Care Nursing, 23*(1), 31–37.

Koestler, A. (1964). *The Act of Creation.* London: Arkana.

Laing, G. (1982). The impact of technology on nursing. *Medical Instrumentation, 16*(5), 241–242.

Locsin, R. (2001). *Advancing Technology, Nursing and Caring.* Westport, CT: Auburn House.

Marck, P. B. (2000). Recovering ethics after 'technics': developing critical text on technology. *Nursing Ethics, 7*, 5–14.

McClure, M. L. (1991). Technology – A driving force for change. *Journal of Professional Nursing, 7*(3), 144.

McConnell, E. A. (1990). The impact of machines on the work of critical care nurses. *Critical Care Nursing Quarterly, 12*(4), 45–52.

McConnell, E. A. (1995). Complexity in selecting health care technology in diverse settings. *Holistic Nursing Practice, 9*, 1–8.

Mitcham, C. (1989). In search of a new relation between science, technology, and society. *Technology and Society, 11*, 409–417.

Mitcham, C. (1994). *Thinking through Technology: The Path between Engineering and Philosophy.* Chicago, IL: The University of Chicago.

Mumford, L. (1934). *Technics and Civilisation.* New York: Harcourt Brace.

Orem, D. (1991). *Nursing: Concepts of Practice.* St Louis, MI: Mosby.

Peacock, J. & Nolan, P. (2000). Care under threat in the modern world. *Journal of Advanced Nursing, 32*(5), 1066–1070.

Pellegrino, E. D. & Thomasma, D. C. (1981). *A Philosophical Basis of Medical Practice.* Oxford: Oxford University Press.

Pelletier, D. (1989). Health care technology: Sharpening the definition and establishing aspects of the social context. *Australian Health Review, 12*(3), 56–64.

Pinch, T. (1991). Book reviews. *Technology and Culture, 32*(10), 1140–1141.

Purcell, C. (1994). *White Heat: People and Technology.* London: BBC Publications.

Reed-Ash, C. (1983). The challenge of technology. *Cancer Nursing, 6*(10), 351.

Reiser, S. J. (1978). *Medicine and the Reign of Technology.* Cambridge: Cambridge University Press.

Reiser, S. J. (1986). Assessment and the technologic present. *International Journal of Technology Assessment in Health Care, 2*, 7–12.

Reverby, S. M. (1987). *Ordered to Care: The Dilemma of American Nursing, 1850–1945.* New York: Cambridge University Press.

Salmon, B. (1969). Nursing in the age of automation. *The New Zealand Nursing Journal, 62*(12), 20–21.

Salmon, B. (1977). Look toward that mountain. *The New Zealand Nursing Journal, 70*(4), 17–21.

Sandelowski, M. (1988). A case of conflicting paradigms: nursing and reproductive technology. *Advances in Nursing Science, 10*(3), 35–45.

Sandelowski, M. (1997). (Ir)Reconcilable differences? The debate concerning nursing and technology. *Image: Journal of Nursing Scholarship, 29*, 169–174.

Sandelowski, M. (2000). *Devices and Desires: Gender, Technology and American Nursing.* Chapel Hill, NC: The University of North Carolina.

Simpson, R. (2002). Nursing informatics: an evolving specialty. *Nursing Economics, 20*(6), 300–301.

Simpson, R. (2003). Today's challenges shape tomorrow's technology, Part 1. *Nursing Management, 34*(10), 16–19.

Simpson, R. L. & Brown, L. N. (1985). High-touch/high-technology computer applications in nursing. *Nursing Administration Quarterly, 9*(4), 62–68.

Simpson, R. L. & Brown, L. N. (1990). How to survive the next decade. *Nursing Management,* *21*(12), 24–25.

Sklair, L. (1971). The sociology of the opposition to science and technology: with special reference to the work of Jacques Ellul. *Comparative Studies in Society and History, 13*(4), 217–235.

Starr, P. (1982). *The Social Transformation of American Medicine.* New York: Basic Books.

Wajcman, J. (1991). *Feminism Confronts Technology.* Oxford: Polity Press.

Walters, A. J. (1994). An interpretative study of the clinical practice of critical care nurses. *Contemporary Nurse, 3,* 21–25.

West, E. (2003). Computers: Do they help or hinder patient care? *Nursing Forum, 38*(1), 29–31.

Wichowski, H. C. (1994). Professional uncertainty: Nurses in the technologically intense arena. *Journal of Advanced Nursing, 19,* 1162–1167.

Wilkin, K. & Slevin, E. (2004). The meaning of caring to nurses: An investigation into the nature of caring work in an intensive care unit. *Journal of Clinical Nursing, 13,* 50–59.

Winner, L. (1977). *Autonomous Technology.* Massachusetts, MA: The MIT Press.

Zwolski, K. (1989). Professional nursing in a technical system. *Image: Journal of Nursing Scholarship, 21*(4), 238–242.

## RECOMMENDED READING

Locsin, R. (ed.) (2001). *Advancing Technology, Caring and Nursing.* Westport, CT: Auburn House.

Sandelowski, M. (2000). *Devises and Desires: Gender, Technology and American Nursing.* Chapel Hill, NC: The University of North Carolina Press.

# Technological Competency as Caring: A Model for Nursing

2

Rozzano Locsin and Alan Barnard

Rozzano Locsin and Alan Barnard

## LEARNING OBJECTIVES

When you have read this chapter, you will be able to:

- Describe the practice of technological competency as caring in nursing

- Explain the concept of 'wholeness of person'

- Describe the process of 'knowing persons' in nursing

- Identify technology-nursing-related situations that influence the relationship between technology, caring and nursing.

## KEY WORDS

- care

- caring

- dynamic

- knowing persons

- nursing

- technology

- technological competency

- theory

- unpredictable

- wholeness

**Vignette:**

Each year, migrant farmers take to the roads travelling a circuit from state to state, harvest to harvest, across the United States. Generations within families travel and work together in the fields, living out their lives in poverty, and being born and dying in the cycle of the harvest. In one South Florida migrant camp during the time of the harvest, a beautiful infant child – a firstborn son – was born to two proud parents. The child was healthy but he was born without arms and legs.

Two weeks after birth, the infant suddenly caught an infection and was rushed to an area hospital for help. Physicians and nurses were stunned: How could they perform the needed technology-based care such as drawing blood for laboratory tests and placing a cuff on the arm or leg to measure blood pressure? Their ability to care for the infant was limited by the technological design of available medical devices. The technology available required a focus on the usual anatomical and physiological composition of a human being; that is the design required a person to have both torso and limbs intact.

Considering this situation and the dependence of many health workers on technology to both assist what they do and define who they are as professionals, the following questions are posited: What is the meaning of being whole, and what does it mean to be complete in the moment?

The purpose of this chapter is to describe technological competency as a practice expressing caring in nursing. To understand this practice it is necessary to have an understanding of three foundational concepts, described as technological competency as caring in nursing; knowing persons as process of nursing; and person whole in the moment. Knowing persons is a deliberate and intentional process of nursing in which human beings are consciously acknowledged as complete, dynamic and unpredictable. Complete refers to the understanding that the composition of human beings (as made up of parts) is not a requisite for knowing persons. Dynamic refers to the ever-changing human phenomena where human beings grow and change. The notion of unpredictability is consistent with an appreciation of each person as a living organism who is continuously changing from one moment to the next. Unpredictability is illustrated in clinical nursing practice where we observe through watchful vigilance for changes in the physiological functioning of patients, for example, watching for changes to arterial blood pressures is crucial in intensive care settings. The act of knowing each person (knowing persons) is a continuous and circuitous activity, in that we regularly return to engage in similar observation and assessment. The nurse seeks to know the nursed in the moment, and because the person is unpredictable, a subsequent desire for knowing is expected and demonstrated as continually assessing and acting with the person. In engaging in this continual activity, the nurse 'knows' the person from moment to moment (see Figure 2.1).

The following example illustrates concepts important to the process of 'knowing person' and the development of technological competency as caring in nursing: 'A nurse examines a child's heart by listening for heart sounds. Doing so using a stethoscope, the nurse "listens" while moving the bell of the stethoscope to strategic areas of the child's chest. The child exclaims, "Why do you keep moving that thing, can't you find my heart?" '

There is simplicity and innocence embedded in the questioning. It is the child's simple images about the situation and those parts of the child's body that are unseen (yet are acknowledged as existing) that create the opportunity for technological competency and a nurse's clear and calm explanation about what he or she was doing. When we seek to know and learn about each patient, as person the practice of nursing is lived meaningfully.

Quite obviously, focusing on a part of the body does not tell us a lot about the whole person or the way the person understands his or her experience. Wholeness of person denotes an appreciation of the 'what' and 'who' of

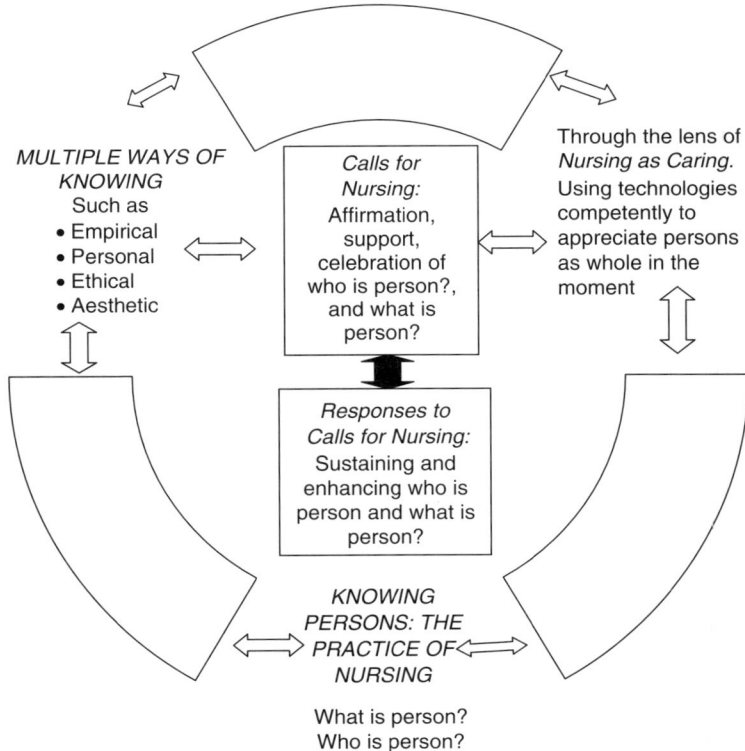

**Figure 2.1** Knowing person as process of nursing. This figure reprinted by permission of Sigma Theta Tan International. All rights reserved.

a 'person'. Interpreting the difference between the 'what' and the 'who' of the person is complex but can be limited by the perspective through which we view and understand the world. For example, 'what' can be expressed as a total summation of a person's physical parts (assimilation/appraising). For some people assessing 'the completeness of a person' might rely only on sensory perception since our sensors (vision, hearing, touch, smell and taste) can obtain a range of data about physical, psychological and physiological well-being. This assessment can, however, tells us little about the person in terms of their emotional and personal well-being. Consider, for example, the 'what' in relation to Frankenstein's monster. The fictitious character was portrayed as committing gruesome crimes in search for his maker and retribution (Shelley, 1969). Whilst Frankenstein's monster has the external characteristics of a human, it exists as a result of its composite parts and is not fully human. The monster was an object with explicit order constructed from the human parts of deceased persons and was made 'alive' to live. The monster wanted connection with his (its) creator and went seeking answers to questions of who he (it) was, to whom he (it) belonged and what was his (its) purpose in being alive (implicit order). The monster found no answers and was rejected by his (its) creator and responded with anger and trauma. The monster was seeking meaning and found nothingness.

When seeking to know a person as whole you must seek to know the relation between both the 'what' and 'who' of the person. In the case of the infant born without arms and legs, he is a human who is whole and complete in the moment, dynamic and unpredictable, with hopes, dreams and aspirations. If you adopt this perspective for all persons, you have opportunity to know the person. You must seek to acknowledge persons as whole. Such an acknowledgment compels nursing – as a practice profession – to invest in and support the use of typical and non-traditional nursing intervention and thinking to affirm, celebrate and support the wholeness of persons. In 'knowing persons' the nurse must seek to understand how each person is complete and whole in the moment.

## 2.1 Completeness in the moment:
## Pieces and wholes

One of the ways that nurses can best demonstrate 'knowing person' is by responding to a person's own descriptions of what matters most to him or her. What is important to a patient is what the nurse 'ought' to know (Allen, 2004). 'Knowing person' in this way provides opportunity for further empowerment for each patient and nurse to selectively, or wholly, participate in the care believed to be most meaningful, beneficial and important. It opens up for us a way to know the patient fully as a person.

In seeking to appreciate whole persons, a limited insight based only on a summation of physical parts is highlighted to be inadequate. In 'wholeness' of a person in the 'moment', the person is whole despite his or her physical presentation. Wholeness in the moment was similarly described by Husserl as an appreciation of wholes and parts that provides two foci: whole as reflective of 'pieces', and whole as reflective of 'moments' (Schultz & Cobb-Stevens, 2004).

This distinction between 'pieces' and 'moments' both expressing the abstract concept of 'whole' helps us to explain those aspects of human beings that are popularly understood by their nature to be made up of their anatomical parts. The understanding that a 'whole cannot exist without its parts' is a consistent reminder of philosophy so typical of a medical model of health in which an appreciation of wholeness is marginalised by a conception that each human being is only a collection of composite 'pieces'. There is recognition that whole is reflective of pieces but there is often a lack of recognition of whole to be reflective of moment. For example, it might be commonplace in your work environment to hear language describing persons as 'the amputee in bed seven'. Knowing the person 'in the moment' is integral to an understanding of persons. Four theoretical explanations assist to describe and explain persons as whole and complete in the moment. The theoretical explanations are person as whole; wholeness of person; person in her/his wholeness; and whole person. Table 2.1 summarises their similarity and difference.

Given that various conceptual descriptions of persons and their wholeness exist in the literature (Boykin & Schoenhofer, 2001; Newman, 1997, 1999; Parse, 1997) the concepts of wholeness and person are appreciated as formative and deserve clarification. Wholeness as an essential focus and practice of nursing

**Table 2.1** The concept of wholeness: Definitions and focus of knowing

| Concepts/terms | Definition | Focus of knowing |
|---|---|---|
| *Wholeness of person* | A person who is a composite of parts, whose completeness is dependent upon the anatomical presence of the part and its complete functioning. Also, the person can be known through the parts | The focus is the wholeness of the person |
| *Person as whole in the moment* | As a whole person characterised by his/her being complete. It is the condition of being whole that matters most. How this wholeness is attained, sustained or maintained dictates the completeness of the person. It is the condition of wholeness and the focus of knowing | The focus is the person in his/her wholeness in the moment. |
| *Persons in their wholeness* | As persons are known in their wholeness, often understood as composed of parts because of their dependency on the parts that make up their whole being. They are appreciated and made known through their completeness. This concept is often interchangeably linked with 'wholeness of persons' | The focus is the person in his/her wholeness |
| *Whole person* | As a whole person who can be known as complete, not needing any fixing, or to be made complete again, regardless of the parts, dependency on his/her parts or characteristics of his/her formation as a whole | The focus is the person in his/her wholeness |

is novel, particularly the view of 'person wholeness in the moment'. The concept is different from the conceptual statements of 'wholeness of person' or 'persons in their wholeness'. An application of the concept of 'person wholeness' is described in the Florida Atlantic University College of Nursing (www.fau.edu/nursing) philosophy of nursing, in which the focus of nursing is nurturing the 'wholeness of persons and environment through caring'. Boykin and Schoenhofer (2001) describe wholeness as the momentary encounter of sharing between the nurse and the patient. Wholeness can be appreciated as a momentary condition because persons are unpredictable.

A primary focus of nursing practice is to 'know persons' (Locsin, 2005a). The story of the infant without upper and lower limbs can illustrate this focus. The infant is whole – a person born without limbs but born as he was made – and complete as a person. If we perceive the child to be less of a person because he has 'different parts', we are seeking to normalise the person and conform him to something other than how he was born. The infant is a living and functioning human being, a person who is whole and complete in the moment.

## 2.2 Wholeness of persons and technological competency

When exposed to novel or unusual situations, technological competency as caring is a challenge to your nursing talent and tests your ability to adapt technology in appropriate and purposeful ways so that it assists you to know the person more fully as complete and whole in the moment. Technology is designed for the 'majority' and is revealed often to be inflexible whenever exposed to a unique application(s). In the vignette at the beginning of the chapter, physicians and nurses were concerned mostly about how they can perform their usual and necessary technological interventions such as withdrawing venous blood to perform laboratory tests and measuring blood pressure, which relies usually on using technology such as a sphygmomanometer attached to a limb. The concern and potential inability to respond quickly and appropriately to the clinical presentation of the child supports the reality of our technological dependency (Sandelowski, 1993). An example of the ways technological competency as caring could be expressed in this situation might relate to establishing priorities in care, determining alternative ways to monitor the child's progress, calmly being with the child and family, clinically assessing the child in alternative ways and consulting with evidence to plan future care.

### The process of nursing

A process of nursing focused on knowing of persons is of value for all nurses and can be integral to the health and well-being of persons. Knowing a person increases the likelihood of quality care and enhances the legitimacy of nursing as a professional practice. Understanding completeness in which the focus and understanding of the person is in relation to his or her pattern of wholeness is explained in Table 2.2, which provides descriptions and definitions of processes of nursing.

**Table 2.2** Processes of nursing and their descriptions and definitions

| Processes of nursing | Descriptions/definitions |
| --- | --- |
| *Knowing person wholeness* | A process in which the focus of nursing practice is to know who the person is, and to understand the person through his/her constitution |
| *Knowing the wholeness of person* | A process of nursing founded on the appreciation of person as a composite of parts that make the person whole, and that knowing the parts as a focus of nursing practice is a way to understand the person |
| *Knowing person* | A process of nursing practice grounded in the understanding that the person is whole regardless of parts, and ought to be known as such |

The concepts of person and wholeness are formative constructs in these processes of nursing. They are constructs critical to understanding the basis for legitimate person-centred nursing practice, discipline formation and professionalism. From a wholeness perspective, the appropriate practice of nursing is 'knowing persons in their wholeness' (see Table 2.2). Wholeness is understood as the *completeness of persons* as determined by the combination of their explicit and implicit order and should not be dependent on social norms or pre-conceived notions of physical and mental normality.

**'Knowing person' as process of nursing**

The vignette about the infant of immigrant workers born without extremities seeks to highlight the concept of completeness of persons regardless of expected cultural or human norms and also exposes one of the challenges of technology in health care because it expects universality and sameness in order to be most efficient. The person did not have the same physical presentation as me and possibly you, but was complete with respect to the way he was formed as a person.

Knowing person as process of nursing is synonymous with commonplace approaches to theory-based nursing practice; that is, nursing practice guided by theories of nursing. Although nursing philosophical and conceptual frameworks are not universally accepted or perhaps understood (Kikuchi, 1997), 'the nursing literature seems to illustrate that the practice of nursing is increasingly being grounded in an explicit grand nursing theory' (Boykin, et al., 2005. p. 15). One such theory of nursing is *Nursing as Caring: A Model for Transforming Practice* (Boykin & Schoenhofer, 2001). Guiding this theory as a model for transforming practice are the following assumptions:

- To be human is to be caring.

- Persons are caring by virtue of their humanness.

- Nursing is nurturing persons, living, caring and growing in caring (Boykin & Schoenhofer, 2001. p. 23).

'Knowing person' as process of nursing demands a conscious and deliberate acknowledgement of persons as whole and complete in the moment. Health care environments remain dependent increasingly on technology, and this dependency has led to a tendency to focus our attention on health care aspects. In these environments, 'technological competency as caring in nursing' is an appropriate model of practice (Locsin, 2001, 2005b), as care is guided by the process of 'knowing persons' even when using technology. Foundational requisites provide structure to this process:

- the understanding of persons as whole and complete in the moment;

- knowing persons as a process of nursinge; and

- technological competency as an expression of caring in nursing.

They are the basis for knowing persons as an evolving practice of nursing. The approach to practice does not require a nurse to only prescribe a process or procedure of care that, in turn, leads to merely tasks and the potential objectification of the patient. 'Knowing person' is meaningfully lived as the continuous knowing of persons from moment to moment. This process of nursing is a deliberate, conscious and intentional recognition of the 'what' and 'who' of a person, one who is whole and complete in the moment (Boykin & Schoenhofer, 2001).

By engaging in this approach to practice, 'knowing' comprises all nursing activities that might include many technologies and include, for example, digital images on a screen, in order for nurses and the health care team to come to know the patient. Nursing as a professional practice and a discipline of knowledge (Boykin & Schoenhofer, 2001) endorses the value of the nurse and patient knowing each other as persons in the moment. 'Coming to know' the other is a purposeful and intentional act of mutual recognition. Establishing ways and means to understand the person, even when care is mediated by the use of technologies, transforms information derived from technology about a specific 'part' of a person into a more complete knowing of the person as whole in the moment. By committing to this process, 'knowing person' is supported through technological competency as caring in nursing.

## Framework for knowing person

What does it mean for you to know the process of knowing person? The process involves continuous collection and verification of data in order to assist you to understand the person as whole and complete in the moment and is evidenced through competent use of technology and meaningful engagement with the individual. Competent care includes appropriate inclusion of technologies that accord with a persons needs, knowledge and skills sufficient to provide evidence-based and thoughtful care, and ongoing skills in clinical judgement that allow you to modify care as conditions change.

In knowing the person, the nurse uses all possible means for the collection, analysis and interpretation of the person's calls for nursing and seeks to engage in a complete and competent implementation of responses. These activities assist you to continuously know the person as whole and complete in the moment. Nursing is a knowledgeable practice informed by a habit of practical reasoning, clinical judgement, compassion and responsibility, and according to Swanson (1993) is characterised by listening, knowing, being with, enabling and maintaining belief. It is supposed to be a knowledgeable and dynamic process that strives to inhibit objectification of the person, and advances the opportunity for each person to be a participant in his or her care despite their vulnerability and need to seek nursing. Daniel (1998) explains that you should 'work to ameliorate vulnerability' (p. 191) and reminds us that 'vulnerable individuals seek nursing care, and nurses seek those who are vulnerable' (p. 192). The following activities exemplify the process of knowing and responding to the uniqueness of persons:

- designing a care plan in which participation in caring is a key principle;
- implementation and ongoing evaluation of the suitability of care (a simultaneous exercise of conjoining relationships crucial to knowing persons by using nursing technologies);
- verifying knowledge of person through continuous data collection; and
- including only those technologies that appropriately meet the care needs and desires of the person.

'Knowing [in] nursing means knowing in the realms of personal, ethical, empirical and aesthetic – all at once' (Boykin & Schoenhofer, 2001, p. 6). This continuous and circular process of knowing highlights the ever-changing, dynamic, cyclical nature of nursing practice. Knowledge about the patient is derived from assessment, intervention, evaluation and further assessment, to continually inform you about the patient. Similarly the patient as a person should also have opportunity to know the nurse (you).This knowing is in part informed by the knowledge that persons are unpredictable. We simultaneously conceal and reveal ourselves as persons from moment to moment. The nurse can only know a patient fully in situated moments, and knowing occurs only when the patient and nurse do not conceal from each other important and necessary aspects of each other's experience. For example, in providing discharge instructions to a patient with diabetes mellitus, the nurse provides the patient with textbook information about food exchanges. Not knowing the patient's food preferences or family traditions of food preparation, may poorly encourage the patient to strive to understand. However, in 'knowing the patient' by assessing and seeking to know the patient's cultural and psycho-social needs, the nurse presents himself/herself as genuinely interested and able to know 'who' the patient is, and in turn the patient can appreciate the nurse being genuinely interested in his well-being.

We advocate that you should practice nursing from a theoretical perspective rather than from just tradition, obedience to instructions and directions, or processes of nursing that are derived from existing theories of nursing that continue to dictate, even often prescribe, how you the nurse should function. Contrary to popular belief, theoretical insight can benefit your care and practice. By knowing persons as a foundation to practice, the mediation of technologies in nursing care provides you with an avenue towards expert nursing, along with the realisation that with technologies you can know the person more fully and acknowledge his or her wholeness. Technologies can only detect the anatomical, physiological, chemical and biological conditions of the patient. Knowing both the 'what' and 'who' of persons affirms the fact that people are more than simply physiological-chemical and anatomical beings.

Knowing persons is a framework for you to understand the person as the focus of nursing in even the most technologically intensive environments. Knowing persons as a process of nursing is a different approach to nursing theory in that there is no ideal prescription or direction provided for your nursing; rather, there is the healthy appreciation of the benefits and foundations of an informed practice that is enhanced by a commitment to caring. The use of technologies for nursing is a consequence of the ongoing demand for nursing action and proficiency of practice. There is no letting up since technologies are a part of the bulk of functional activities we nurses are expected to perform in clinical settings. Hospital nursing is dominated by practice founded on skilful application of technologies in patient treatment.

The process of knowing persons emphasises that the focus of care is the patient, not as an object of care, but as a participant in their care. Technological competency as caring in nursing provides you with thinking skills and potential for independence to critically decide modes of action that allow for appreciation of the whole person. As participants in care, and when patients allow you to 'enter their world', each patient will declare the best possible ways they want to be cared for at any moment. Sometimes this may only require you to be physically present in the moment.

Persons require continuous knowing because of the dynamic/changing nature of being human. When patients participate in their care, they free the nurse from imposing care that they otherwise may not want. Continuous knowing by the nurse results from the contention that in knowing we desire to know more about 'who is' and 'what is' the person. The process encourages affirmation, support and celebration of the hopes, dreams and aspirations of each human being.

Figure 2.1 illustrates the dynamic process of knowing a person through technological competency as caring in nursing. In knowing a person, calls for nursing are heard by the nurse to affirm, support and celebrate persons as whole in the moment. Responses to these calls will relate to the need to sustain the person as whole. This relationship is dynamic as illustrated by the two-way arrows complementing the process of 'calls and responses'. In 'knowing', ways of appraising persons are employed through an awareness of nursing as caring (Boykin & Schoenhofer, 2001), and knowing persons is achieved through technological competency in nursing practice. The nurse and the person nursed live out a meaningful relationship – both seeking to know each other in the moment.

## 2.3 Final reflection

There is a growing need and demand for nursing practice that is based on an authentic desire to know human beings as persons. To meet these needs and demands nursing has to develop ways for each nurse to use technologies to address calls for nursing and come to know the person as whole in the moment. The following poem by Sheila Carr (1999) highlights the experience when these calls and responses as an expression of technological competency as caring in nursing have not been met by a nurse. Expression of technological competence can assist in the goals of persons being realised. With a genuine intention to care, the nurse is challenged to make a commitment to use every creative, imaginative, available and innovative way to appreciate and celebrate the person's living and growing as a human being.

INTENSIVE CARE

Did you see nurse that you can know me –
The part that is me, my mind and soul is in my eyes
These tubes that are everywhere – that is not me.
The one in my throat is the worst of all –
Now my whole being, the essence of me I
must reflect through my hands but they are tied down
but did you realize that it is uncomfortable for me
or through my eyes and you do not notice them –
except once today during my bath.
You speak to me and look at the tubes –
Don't you know my thoughts are all over my face
Don't you realize your thoughts are on your face –
In your touch and your tone of voice.
I wrote a request on paper you said 'I'll take care
of it for you' your tone said 'Why can't this
woman do anything for herself?'
You positioned your hand to count my pulse but I
can't say you touched me – you wouldn't hold my hand that I may touch you.
You walked in for the first time today with a grin on your face
but your mouth is now tight and you grimaced a lot as you bathed me.
Don't you see nurse that you can know me – I'm not
a chart or tubes of medication, monitors or all
the other things you look at so intensely – I'm
more than that, I'm scared – just look in my eyes.

**Sheila Carr**

**LEARNING ACTIVITIES**

1. Discuss the relationship between technological competency as caring in nursing and knowing persons as a process of nursing.

2. Identify three occasions you have experienced where understanding the whole person would have improved care.

3. In small groups list three technology-nursing-related situations. In the larger group report, formulate an accumulative list of these technology-nursing situations based on all the responses from groups and rank their relative priority.

## References

Allen, D. (2004). Re-reading nursing and re-writing practice: Towards an empirically based reformulation of the nursing mandate. *Nursing Inquiry, 11*(4), 271–283.

Boykin, A. & Schoenhofer, S. (2001). *Nursing as Caring: A Model for Transforming Practice*. New York: Jones & Bartlett, National League for Nursing Press.

Boykin, A., Bulfin, S., Schoenhofer, S., Baldwin, J. & McCarthy, D. (2005). Living caring in practice: The transformative power of the theory of Nursing as Caring. *International Journal for Human Caring, 9*(3), 115–119.

Carr, S. (1999). Intensive Care. *Nightingale Songs: A Forum for Nursing*. Christine E. Lynn College of Nursing. www.fau.edu/nursing.

Daniels, L. (1998). Vulnerability as a key to authenticity. *Image: Journal of Nursing Scholarship, 30*(2), 191–192.

Kikuchi, J. (1997). Clarifying the nature of conceptualizations about nursing. *Canadian Journal of Nursing Research, 29*(1), 97–110.

Locsin, R. (2001). Practicing nursing: Technological competency as caring in nursing. In R. Locsin (ed.), *Advancing Technology, Caring, and Nursing*. Westport, CT: Auburn House.

Locsin, R. (2005a). Technological competency as caring, and the practice of knowing persons as whole. In M. Parker (ed.). *Nursing Theories and Nursing Practice* (2nd edn.). Philadelphia, PA: F. A. Davis.

Locsin, R. (2005b). Knowing persons as a framework for nursing. In R.C. Locsin (ed.), *Technological Competency as Caring in Nursing: A Model for Practice*. Indianapolis, IN: Center Nursing Press, Sigma Theta Tau International.

Newman, M. (1997). Experiencing the whole. *Advances in Nursing Science, 20*(1), 34–39.

Newman, M. (1999). The rhythm of relating in a paradigm of wholeness. *Image: Journal for Nursing Scholarship, 31*(3), 227–229.

Parse, R. (1997). The human becoming theory: The was, is, and will be. *Nursing Science Quarterly, 10*, 80–87.

Sandelowski, M. (1993). Toward a theory of technology dependency. *Nursing Outlook, 41*(1), 36–42.

Schultz, G. & Cobb-Stevens, R. (2004). Husserl's theory of wholes and parts and the methodology of nursing research. *Nursing Philosophy, 5*, 216–223.

Shelley, M. (1969). *Frankenstein: Or the Modern Prometheus*. New York: Oxford University Press.

Swanson, K. (1993). Nursing as informed caring for the well-being of others. *Image: Journal of Nursing Scholarship, 25*(4), 352–357.

## RECOMMENDED READING

Locsin, R. (2005). *Technological Competency as Caring in Nursing: A Model for Practice*. Indianapolis, IN: Sigma Theta Tau International Press.

Locsin, R. (ed.) (2001). *Advancing Technology, Caring and Nursing*. Westport, CT: Auburn House.

Schultz, G. & Cobb-Stevens, R. (2004). Husserl's theory of wholes and parts and the methodology of nursing research. *Nursing Philosophy, 5*, 216–223.

# Intensive Care and Technology: Neonatal and Adult Nursing Practice

3

## Deborah Raines and Kathryn Keller

When you have read this chapter, you will be able to:

- Outline key issues in the development of nurses role in intensive care

- Explain the relations between intensive care nursing, technology and caring

- Reflect upon the advantages of applying frameworks to assist nursing practice in adult and neonatal nursing environments

- Discuss important advantages and strategies for enhancing human focused care in technology-intensive care environments

## KEY WORDS

- caring

- intensive care nursing

- neonatal

- practice frameworks

- technology assessment

## 3.1 Technology and nursing practice

In the past 50 years, health care has experienced a proliferation of advances in scientific knowledge and technology. These advances have had a profound impact on the care of individuals across the lifespan. The acceptance of high-tech units in the health care system has led to the expectation that high technology can cure the most acutely ill individual and save individuals at each extreme of the lifespan continuum. The focus of this chapter is the interface of technology and nursing care in two specific high-tech areas, the Neonatal Intensive Care Unit (NICU) and the Adult Intensive Care Unit (ICU).

Neonatal intensive care units are defined by the American Academy of Pediatrics (1980) as nurseries that provide for constant and continuous care of the critically ill newborn. Modern neonatal intensive care has a relatively short history. Early descriptions of intensive care for newborns were often discussed in conjunction with adult intensive care. However, during the 1960s the scope of neonatal care expanded and the area of concern evolved from acceptance of the death of premature infants to efforts concentrating on rescuing these infants with technology (American Academy of Pediatrics, 2002). This change in perspective has played a major and definitive role in the improved survival of low birth weight and premature infants. Each day in the United States 1,300 babies are born prematurely and a number of others are born sick or with complications resulting from pregnancy or birth. These are the children who make up the NICU population (March of Dimes, 2005).

The NICU of today provides the machinery to save infants at younger and younger gestational ages and at lower and lower birth weights. These advances in technology have also resulted in improved capacities in the diagnosis and treatment of disease and disability. These technologies include, but are not limited, to prenatal diagnosis, intrauterine surgery, mechanical ventilation, ECMO (extra-corporeal membrane oxygenation) and the use of pharmacologic agents such as artificial surfactant to assist the infant in making the transition to extra-uterine existence when a pathologic condition or prematurity make the circumstances of survival less than optimal.

Meanwhile, the evolution of technology in the adult Intensive Care Unit has progressed into its fifth decade. ICUs originated in the 1960s and at that time nurses were taught to defibrillate, perform peritoneal dialysis, administer mechanical rotating tourniquets and monitor the ventilator and electrocardiograph rhythms (Burrell, 1969). Technology was firmly established in this era and the evolution of this technology has been impressive. The list of technological devices has grown to include care of intra-aortic balloon pumps, pulmonary artery catheters, arterial monitoring devices, chest-tube systems, central lines, left ventricular assist devices, programmable trans-venous pacemakers and bedside haemodialysis systems. These technologies have necessitated in depth, educational endeavours. Traditionally, education has centred primarily on the theory and workings of the device. The associated caring that connects with the person has always been present but has not received the same amount of formal education. Nurses have had almost 50 years to develop formalised systems of care in intensive care settings that would allow for nurses to interact with the person while simultaneously manipulating the accompanying technology.

Technology is not intrinsically good or bad, but its beneficial or harmful effects will depend on how we use or apply it. A major challenge for us is that scientific advances are occurring at a greater rate than our ability to evaluate their usefulness in the practice environment. The introduction of high-tech devices in the health care setting has led to a deeply ingrained pattern of perpetual production and consumption that constitutes an invisible but powerful device for the fundamental shaping of our expectations. For example, in a study focused on the values of parents of low birth weight infants, a number of participants initially identified a direct link between the presence of the technology in the NICU and the infant's survival (Raines, 1998). However, with the passage of time, the recognition of technology as a device became evident:

> Things are more frail than I expected ... things could go wrong because it's not all machines where you just stick in the fluid and they grow and out they go ... The monitors give a warning that something may be wrong ... but the need for human decision and competence make it a very dangerous place. (p. 44)

There is no doubt that the main reason for the vast improvement in the quality of our lives in the last century is due to the great technological advances that have taken place. The phenomenal increase in the standards of living that occurred in the industrialised world (and to a lesser extent in other countries) following the scientific revolution of the 1800s was a direct consequence of the invention, improvements and spread of technological know-how. Needless to say, the same improvements have occurred in the health care setting. In the 1960s we realised that we had the knowledge and tools necessary to sustain and cure even the most critically ill patients, and the intensive care units were born. As a result, critical care nurses have witnessed amazing advances in their professional environment. These technological advancements have had many implications for nursing practice.

## 3.2 Technology assessment

Professionally, nurses should not blindly accept every technological innovation to arrive in clinical practice. Not every technological 'innovation' will, at the end of the day, prove to be beneficial, and, as such, we owe it to our patients to thoroughly evaluate and scrutinise the use of new technology. High-tech care results in both increased survival and increased costs. In addition, intensive care becomes more expensive as it is employed in increasingly marginal cases. The worth of a life saved however is ultimately a value judgement involving ethical and social considerations. The result from 'cost effectiveness studies alone can't guide decisions regarding who should receive care' (Herdman et al., 1987). Nurses, who are the primary users of many technologies, are in prime positions to determine the influences and potential harmful effects. In this regard, nurses' input is invaluable when it is needed to assess technology.

No one who works in the ICU would deny the benefits that technology has brought to our field. Yet, technology assessment needs to be built into our systems as a matter of priority and expectation. Marsden (1991) states that critical care nurses must assess new and expanding technologies as they are introduced into the ICU and prepare to cope with the changes they bring. She further states that when ICU nurses assess technology, they usually ask straightforward questions about its safety, efficacy and benefit to the patient. Many new technologies reach the ICU before their efficacy and impact are fully known. ICU nurses need to assess new technologies and be prepared to design the protocols of care needed to cope with the accompanying changes to practice.

One of the difficult issues that frequently arise in the ICU is the application of advanced technology to sustain the life of terminally ill cases. This is one of the main areas of dissatisfaction and frustration for ICU nurses. These situations involve many different dilemmas such as ethical issues, differences of opinion among health care givers, lack of advance directives from the patient, unrealistic expectations from family members and difficulty in accurately predicting life-altering outcomes. These conflicts are a direct result of technology advancement and impact nursing care. Advances have been made in the past several years, such as encouraging patients to have a living will, developing tools to more accurately predict mortality in critically care individuals and the early use of hospice services. One of the most contentious issues arises when the family members insist that 'everything be done' when health care providers know well that the situation is futile. Many times the problem derives from lack of communication. The ICU nurse tends to spend a great deal of time with visiting family and is well positioned to establish a rapport. When the families know that their loved one is being cared for in a skilled and compassionate manner, they will more often than not accept the recommendations of the health care providers with respect to life-supporting measures.

## 3.3   Technologies impact: An ethical perspective

Technological advances are occurring at a rapid rate and are affecting clinical practice before health care professionals are able to develop guidelines or foresee the social and ethical impacts of these interventions. The proliferation of high-tech units has resulted in nurses being confronted with difficult decisions related to the management and care of patients, leading to frustration and uneasiness. The ethical principles foundational to nursing practice are autonomy, confidentiality, veracity, beneficence and justice. However, the application of these principles to daily nursing practice is more complex. The challenge of this situation is intensified in high-tech practice areas since many patients in these environments are unable to decide or participate in treatment decisions. Often decisions are delegated to a third party. Thus the question becomes not only who should be making decisions but also what values are important in guiding these decisions. Decisions reflect the personal/professional values of the individuals involved in the process. Nurses, because of their continuous involvement with the patient and the family, become vital participants in these situations; therefore, their values may profoundly influence their behaviour in the application of ethical principles in the practice setting. An examination of the ethical principles as applied to the high-tech nursing care environment will illustrate the unique challenges faced by the nurse.

The principle of autonomy is based on free acceptance by the patient of the treatment option. A major difficulty in high-tech units is that there is no way to know what the individual would choose in the given situation. In the NICU, the infant not only lacks the ability to communicate but also lacks the life experience and past history for us to fully know the person. They cannot provide a personal set of values and beliefs to influence choices. The infant's autonomy is delegated to a surrogate decision maker. As expected, this would fall normally to the parents who have the authority to decide for the infant, whereas in an adult ICU the individuals whose ability to communicate or participate in decision making is impaired by their condition have a set of personal values and beliefs and life experience and history, but whose knowledge and understanding of their values and beliefs best represent the patient. The best surrogate decision maker for the person can be a difficult question. New family structures and recognition of relationships with others add new dimensions to who should decide for the patient in the adult ICU.

The principles of confidentiality and veracity are closely related to surrogate decision making in that they encompass the issue of who has access to information. The principle of confidentiality is foundational to the provider–patient relationship. However, information sharing about treatment options, outcome, benefits and potential complications are critical to informed decision-making. The principles of confidentiality are also closely intertwined with the patient's relationship with others: does the legal institute of marriage or the social commitment between individuals take precedence in determining one's role and access to information?

The determination of the best interests of the patient is based on quality of life arguments and is related to the principles of non-maleficence. Increasingly health care professionals believe that the value of life for an individual is related to the individual's own perception of the quality of that life. However, high-tech units are making living possible for individuals who in the past would not have a decision to make. But these choices come with positives, negatives and, most significantly, a lot of unknown.

Finally, as a result of today's health care environment, which is typically afflicted with cost containment, staff shortages and limited resources, a discussion of the ethical dimensions of high-tech care requires an examination of the principle of justice: how are beds and hi-tech resources allocated? The question of which treatment is ordinary or expected as a component of nursing care and which is extraordinary are integral to a discussion of the principle of justice.

## 3.4 Evaluation of high-tech care

In health care, the implications of each treatment option are considered based on its potential long-term outcome. The impact of new knowledge, advanced technology, social concerns and economic forces has forced nursing to re-evaluate its historical roots and role in the provision of health care. The technological breakthroughs of the past 50 years have had a dramatic impact on the moral evaluation of health care delivery systems as well as on the discipline of nursing. External evaluation of health care is forcing nurses to be accountable to the consumer, and society as a whole for their choices and behaviours. Nurses are the health care providers with the closest and most prolonged contact with the patient. In these roles as care giver, counsellor, educator and protector, the nurse has a pivotal role in creating a forum in which consistent, sensitive and knowledgeable decision-making care occur.

In neonatal care, the outcome is not immediately evident: an infant is not a finished product. From a physiological point of view the infant continues to grow and develop through childhood and adolescence. It is well documented that a number of systems including the neurological, musculoskeletal and respiratory systems continue to mature following the completion of intrauterine development. The survivors of today's neonatal units are charting an unknown path into the future. What effect will the treatment of today have on the infant's ongoing process of physiological, psychological and emotional development and well-being? The long-term implications of the interventions that made it possible for the individual to survive are unknown. And because of the speedy proliferation of technology and the rapidly changing standard in the realm of peri-natal care, there may never be well-defined outcomes by which to measure risk–benefit ratio of neonatal care.

In adult ICUs the long-term impact on patients surviving serious illness that required prolonged care are relatively unknown. There is little evaluative data on how technological interventions in the ICU impact patients both functionally and cognitively on a long-term basis. Nurses practicing in these areas need to collaborate with practitioners in the home care setting to evaluate the long-term outcomes of high-tech focused care. Examination of the measurable outcome such as morbidity and mortality are important but do not reveal the impact of high-tech care.

## 3.5 Nursing frameworks and technological caring behaviours in neonatal ICU

Neonatal nurses practice in an environment established on the expectation that high-technology neonatal intensive care can save and cure even the tiniest and sickest of infants. According to Guillemin (1982) the values that have driven the expansion of neonatal intensive care are

- the equation of biological life of the foetus/infant with an idealised and full-blown adult identity;
- the espousal of acute care as the solution to health problems;
- the belief in the power of the specialist.

The care of the neonate has been directly and extensively changed by the expansion of the very specialised and highly technically dependent units. The change in the work environment has direct implications for the practice of nurses in the NICU. Nursing has generally followed the lead of medicine: nurses have learned the technical skills and developed the expertise to actively participate in the delivery of neonatal intensive care. However, as a profession based on holistic care for the patients and the family and on the concepts of care, coordination and advocacy, nurses must question the morality of this approach. When parents were asked to prioritise the attribute most desirable in the nurse caring for their neonate, competence and caring were ranked as the highest priorities (Raines, 1998). Unfortunately, the discipline's attention to the professional role and accountability of the nurse in determining the future direction of neonatal care has often been eclipsed by the focus on technological expertise. That is, we spend a lot of time focusing on what 'we have to do', without equal consideration of 'the implications and meaning of our action(s)'.

All the goals of nursing are not scientific: They are moral and are based on the seeking of good. Consequently nursing practice and education seeks often to assimilate not only the scientific and factual knowledge needed to implement hi-tech care found in NICUs but a commitment to provide caring, humane, person-oriented nursing care in an environment of uncertainty. Desirable health care outcomes have been based typically on quantifiable and obvious outcomes such as measures of survival and mortality, changes in lab data or modifications in technical supports. However, the intent of health care outcomes needs to evolve to recognise and accept the process of patient care and the intangible outcomes such as connecting, helping and caring, which typically are part of nursing practice, especially in an environment of uncertainty. Quality patient care requires a combination of medical, social and nursing considerations. The utility of high technology in the neonatal care setting emerges from a sequential interaction between values or internal standards of right and wrong and an assessment of contextual information in each nursing situation. In the NICU, time is critical and gut-level decisions are made sometimes with limited information about immediate and long-term consequences.

Benner (1991) identified ethical demeanour as doing better or worse where better cannot be strictly rule governed or procedural, because it must be guided by situated understanding of particular human concerns. Nurses in the NICU care form a highly vulnerable population. Nurses are the health care providers with the best understanding of the particular human concerns of each individual patient, and as caring professional nurses need to develop proactive, accountable positions, fostering increased sensitivity and receptiveness to individual patient situations and forcing the health care system to look beyond the tangible outcomes and seeking the better outcome for each individual patient.

## 3.6 Nursing frameworks and technological caring behaviours in adult ICU

Caring for people in the high-tech environments in the ICU presents many challenges. The nurse must be familiar with the advanced technology surrounding the person, yet be able to value the humanness, that is the person.

Each piece of technology brought into the ICU environment presents a challenge to the nurses to construct the caring that will accompany the machinery. The word 'caring' as mentioned above should not be confused with the idea of specific technological skill or competency acquisition, but rather the professional caring behaviours the nurse brings to the situation. Roach (2002) has categorised attributes of professional caring into six categories, which are compassion, competence, confidence, conscience, commitment and comportment. These professional attributes of caring are depicted in behaviours such as '... taking the time to be with, checking factual information, identifying and using relevant knowledge, performing technical procedures ...' (Roach, 2002, p. 43).

The attributes acknowledge technological competence, yet emphasise caring characteristics as equally important. Roach best illustrates this by stating, ' ... competence without compassion can be brutal and inhumane, compassion without competence may be no more than a meaningless, if not harmful, intrusion into the life of a person or persons needing help' (Roach, 2002, p. 54). Further to this, Locsin (2005, p. 7) states that 'Often, technological competency is viewed as the opposite of caring. However, these two concepts – traditional caring and technological competency as caring – have a relationship that is critical to nursing practice'.

Locsin explains that technological competency as caring in nursing is a conceptual model that occurs when caring and technology coexist appropriately in nursing. Technological competence as caring is the practice of using technology for the purpose of knowing persons. Critical care nursing is a continuous knowing of persons through the competent use of technologies. Competency with technology is a skilled demonstration of intentional and authentic activities by experienced nurses who practice in environments requiring technological expertise (Locsin, 2005). Portraying knowledgeable caring is the highest form of commitment in giving patient care (Sherwood, 1997). It is through intention that we achieve competence, and through competence we realise confidence. Roach's work in conjunction with Locsin's model offers the critical care nurse insight into how to understand and shape their practice environment.

### Exemplar for caring technological protocols: Neonatal ICU

> Cherry gazed down at the tiny, tiny babies, curled up asleep in their special beds, some of them not much bigger than her two fists. One of them had no fingernails or toenails yet. Another one had no eyelashes yet. It was work for them to even breathe ... . Some of these morsels of humanity might live and some day becomes strong men and women, some might not survive the year. Cherry felt a wave of pity as she looked at the struggling little beings. She thought of their mothers, too. (Wells, 1943)

In the past neonatal nursing care was very different. The main responsibility of the health care professional was to examine the infants and write feeding orders for the premature infants. All premature infants received half-skim milk with carbohydrates added – it was very straightforward. There were no intravenous lines, no ventilators, no ultrasounds and no choice of formula or micronutrient determinations. Laboratory testing was confined to blood counts and capillary glucose measures. Mothers were not allowed to touch or hold these tiniest of infants. Mothers were obligated to view their child through the nursery window, not even being allowed into the nursery environment. Yes, there was infant transport – infants were carried in little animal boxes with a hot water bottle as a source of heat. But whether the tiniest of infants remained at the birth hospital or were transported to another facility, infants weighing less than 1000 grams rarely survived.

Today's NICU is not like a typical nursery with pink and blue frills and clowns and balloons. In the NICU there are bright lights and a variety of machines, tubes and monitors, each emitting its own unique sound and visual signal. Although the sights and sounds of the NICU can be overwhelming, very few are human in nature, and the massiveness of the technology can easily outweigh any human presence. Yet, in the midst of all the technology is an infant in need of nursing care.

A typology of three types of infants is usually found in the NICU: very immature infant, infants with genetically linked syndrome and acutely ill or unstable infants (Raines, 1993). The metamorphosis from premature nursery to special care nursery to neonatal intensive care unit was gradual and parallels the introduction of technology. However, technology alone is not responsible for the decrease in neonatal morbidity and mortality. Nurses occupy a unique role in the care of neonates. Nurses have continuous contact with the infant and responsibility for the implementation of professional standards of nursing care. Nurses come to know the neonate as a unique being and make a commitment to advocate for that being's welfare. As participants in decisions about the use of the available technologies in the care and management of the neonate, the behaviours chosen by the nurse results in care and support essential to the infant's survival and well-being. The competence, commitment, courage and consciousness of the nurse is foundational to one's perception of a situation and the actions or inactions that influence outcomes of the NICU experience and impact individuals, families and society as a whole.

### Exemplar for caring technological protocols: Adult ICU

One of the best exemplars that illustrate the need for incorporating caring behaviours alongside technological competence is the trend to include family to be present during a cardiac resuscitation effort. Picture an adult patient in a high-tech environment who is critically ill. His condition has been deteriorating and his vital signs are unstable. There is a real danger that he could go into a cardiac arrest at any time. A family member is present at the bedside and is aware of the gravity of the situation. The family member has voiced his/her desire to stay during any critical situation. The electrocardiograph (ECG) monitor's alarms begin to sound and nursing personnel quickly enter the room. The ECG monitor shows ventricular fibrillation. The defibrillator is brought to the bedside and a cardiac resuscitation effort begins. The defibrillator requires technological competence, along with intubation knowledge and line insertion. We know that advanced cardiac life support protocols are taking place, yet what are the professional caring behaviours that would allow the nurse to guide a family member through this process? Nursing and medical staff have been highly resistant to this notion. However, the literature reflects a trend towards implementing and evaluating this controversial stance (McGahey, 2002; Albertan & Stafford, 1999). Our paediatric nursing colleagues have been the leaders in refining and implementing this concept. Very few adult ICUs have established a protocol; however, this is not the case in adult emergency departments. A decade ago the Emergency Nurses Association came out in support of family presence programs. They also included a position of family presence during invasive procedures (McGahey, 2002). Adult ICU nurses need to review the work that has been accomplished by these other areas. Developing family presence programs for adult ICUs is necessary work and will guide other caring technological protocols.

## 3.7 Technology interference and caring behaviours

Another variable that affects caring behaviours in the ICU high-tech environment is 'treatment interference'. Treatment interference is the disruption or self-removal of technological devices (Happ, 1998, 2000). The self-removal of an arterial line or endotracheal tube can have immediate and disastrous results. Nurses are responsible for maintaining the effectiveness of technological devices. Nurse researchers have begun to study this occurrence and to identify interventions. Nursing responsibilities include skilful assessment of patients' cognitive status, mobility, strength and trustworthiness. Interventions that have been identified are repeated explanations, distraction and sedation; assessing the discontinuation status of the device; watchful family members; and physical restraints. Whereas nurses have always maintained the function of technological devices, additionally nurses are almost exclusively responsible for protecting these devices from dislodgement or damage. This is an inherent nursing responsibility in the ICU. The concept of treatment interference directly influences professional caring behaviours in that restraints and sedation are often employed to safeguard technology.

One of the responsibilities of the ICU nurse is to ensure that important devices are not tampered with by 'others'. Many patients are less than alert either because of illness or pharmacotherapeutics. It is a natural tendency to try and pull out devices that are perceived as foreign or invading the body. For example, the unintentional removal of a life-sustaining technology such as ventilator tubing has dire consequences. In this context, the use of restraints has become a necessary evil. Although communicating to the person why they should not tamper with devices is the first intervention, many times alertness will vary throughout the day. Often the patient is sedated. The nurse cannot always rely on explanation and a family member at the bedside. In fact, some family members may not want the responsibility of safeguarding devices. The use of soft restraints is a common occurrence in an advanced technological environment. When this occurs, the need for a caring presence is paramount.

This is an area that needs realistic and practical protocols that will provide a caring environment, yet ensure the safety of the person connected to the technological device.

## 3.8 Final reflection: The future of technology and ICU nursing

Technology is a benefit and a burden. Technology forces us to understand new concepts, to approach old problems in novel ways, to master the use of new devices and to learn to interpret the results. In this regard, we each must be committed to constant educational renewal in the ICU. The role of the ICU nurse is a dynamic one because of the constant challenge of mastering new technology. With acquired knowledge and skills come increased accountability, respectability and greater autonomy. There is much more to nursing than the implementation of scientific knowledge and technology. In fact, how care is provided is at the core of what nursing is all about. Professional caring attributes are what distinguishes nurses from the other health professionals. A caring nurse knows the importance of providing comfort and reassurance to patients and families alike. By opening lines of communication, nurses can allay fears and lessen the anxiety associated with the ICU experience. A gentle touch and a reassuring, calming voice can be extraordinarily beneficial to a patient or family member who is terrified of the ICU experience. The challenge for the ICU nurse, now and in the future, is to find the balance between the use of technologies and professional ethical behaviours.

### LEARNING ACTIVITIES

1. In small groups discuss strategies for enhancing human focused care in high-technology environments. Can these strategies be used also in less intensive environments? In a larger group, provide an example of non-human focused care and explain how you would implement your strategy.

2. Write down an approach to integrate nursing frameworks in clinical practice to advance care in adult and neonatal environments.

3. In the group form two teams and debate the assertion that 'technology should not be the focus of nursing practice'.

## References

Albertan, J. W. & Stafford, H. (1999). Resusitation and family presence: Implications for nurses in critical care areas. *Advanced Clinical Nurse*, 3, 11–19.

American Academy of Pediatrics (2002). *Guide for Perinatal Care* (5th edn.). Elk Grove Village, IL: AAP.

Benner, P. (1991). The role of experience, narrative, and community in skilled ethical comportment. *Advances in Nursing Science, 14*(2), *1–21.*

Burrell, Z. & Burrell, L. (1969). *Intensive Nursing Care.* Saint Louis, MI: CV Mosby.

Guillemin, J. H. (1982). The price of medical heroics. *Society,* Jan/Feb, 31–38.

Happ, M. B. (1998). Treatment Interference in acutely and critically ill adults. *American Journal of Critical Care, 7*(3), 224–235.

Herdman, R. C., Behney, C. J., Wagner, J. L. & Ehrenhaft, P. M. (1987). *Neonatal Intensive Care for Low Birthweight Infants: Cost and Effectiveness.* (OTA-HCS-38). Washington, DC: United States Printing Office.

Locsin, R. (2005). *Technological Competency as Caring in Nursing: A Model for Practice.* Indianapolis, IN: Center Nursing Press, Sigma Theta Tau International.

March of Dimes (2005) Prematurity acts. http://www.marchofdimes.com/prematurity/5415_8612.asp [Accessed 25 September 2005.]

Marsden, C. (1991). Technology assessment in critical care. *Heart & Lung, 20*(1), 93–94.

McGahey, P. (2002). Family presence during pediatric resuscitation: A focus on staff. *Critical Care Nurse, 22*(6), 29–34.

Raines, D. A. (1998). Values of mothers of low birth weight infants in the NICU. *Neonatal Network, 17*(4), 41–46.

Raines, D. A. (1993). Deciding what to do when the patient can't speak. *Neonatal Network, 12*(6), 43–48.

Roach, M. S. (2002). *Caring: The Human Mode of Being* (2nd rev. edn.). Ottawa, A Canadian Hospital Association Press.

Sherwood, G. (1997). Patterns of caring: the healing connection of interpersonal harmony. *International Journal for Human Caring, 1*(1), 30–38.

Wells, H. (1943). *Cherry Ames Student Nurse.* New York: Grosset and Dunlap.

## RECOMMENDED READING

Barnard, A. & Sandelowski, M. (2001). Technology and humane nursing care: A(n) (ir)reconcilable or invented difference? *Journal of Advanced Nursing, 34*(3), 367–375.

Sandelowski, M. (2000). *Devises and Desires: Gender, Technology and American Nursing.* Chapel Hill, NC: The University of North Carolina Press.

Timmermans, S. (1997) High touch in high tech: The presence of relatives and friends during resuscitative efforts. *Scholarly Inquiry for Nursing Practice, 11,* 153–168.

# Ethical Implications of Technology on the Patient–Nurse Interaction

Susan Beidler and Susan Chase

## LEARNING OBJECTIVES

When you have read this chapter, you will be able to:

- Describe ethical considerations in the use of communication technology.
- Identify the role of laws and codes of ethics in protecting patient information.
- Identify international mechanisms for determining credible e-health-related Internet sites.
- Discuss the role of nursing as a patient advocate in emerging tele-health-related policy.

## KEY WORDS

- communication
- confidentiality
- ethics
- health policy
- nursing
- patient–nurse interaction
- technology

## 4.1  Introduction

The daily practice of nursing has been altered by the demands of technology, which commands nursing's commitment, attention and time (Barnard, 2000). The intrinsic value of technology as either *good* or *bad* is ultimately determined by the nurse's view of its impact on the patient. Advanced information technology has been identified as the solution to problems of human suffering by providing access to care not otherwise available (Gallagher, 2000). While some nurses view the use of technology as advancing the profession and improving social and professional harmony, others have viewed it as a destruction of nursing's basic core. The basic core of nursing has historically been identified as the nurse–patient relationship (King, 1981; Peplau, 1987, 1992). This relationship has been identified as a patient–nurse covenant (Beidler, 2002), which reflects the notion of a promise made between the patient and nurse to work together towards common goals. Another way of addressing this relationship is that the basic core of nursing is the commitment to advocate for and provide the best possible care for all patients. Regardless of technological advancements and settings, nurses in relationship with patients promote, maintain and restore health and wellness.

In this chapter, the term *relationship* has been substituted with the term *interaction* for several reasons. In her effort to address the complexity of nursing, Meleis (1997) issued a call for paradigmatic pluralism or a variety of viewpoints in nursing and voiced the need for a theory about interactions. Morse (1991), similarly valuing this theoretical need, described patterns of relating as context-dependent with purposeful interaction. Hagerty and Patusky (2003) analysed assumptions inherent in contemporary theoretical and empirical literature on the nurse–patient relationship and also proposed an alternate framework, identified as the nurse–patient *interaction* that was more congruent with the current health care environment. Thus, the term *relationship* has been substituted with the term *interaction* for the purpose of providing a more conceptual fit with emerging theories. The transposition of *nurse* and *patient* from *nurse–patient* to *patient–nurse* also reflects the post-modern view of the patient as the dominant focus in the interaction.

This chapter reviews the ways in which technology exercises power to change essential nursing functions. A neutral view which releases technology from any intrinsic value of worth or worthlessness must be addressed (Barnard, 1997). As a result of a perception of neutrality of technology, the potential misuse of technology creates legal and ethical concerns, some of which are highlighted in this chapter. Ethical implications of technology as it is used to communicate with patients, to provide health information and to provide health care interventions are necessary to consider when utilising current and developing technologies in health care delivery.

## 4.2  Protection of patient information – ethical implications

The use of technology to supplant or enhance communication is not a new phenomenon. Communication technology in one of its earliest forms was the telephone. Inasmuch as nursing is a communication-based profession, the telephone was used to enhance patient care. Newer communication technologies, such as Internet-based electronic mail and videoconferencing also enhance patient care, but not without ethical considerations. Of utmost concern is the protection of patient information.

## The Internet

The Internet influences a wide range of health care activities, such as purchasing health-related products and services, ordering prescription medications, obtaining consumer information services, accessing personal health records, managing personal health information, communicating between health care providers and patients, medical advisement and diagnosis, and participating in support groups (Maddox, 2002). The Internet has had an unprecedented impact on the communication of health information. Millions of consumers worldwide are using the Internet to obtain quality health information, which makes this form of technology an important new tool for improving health care. Information that was only available to health professionals by attending conferences and reading professional journals is now available to patients as immediately as it is presented, published or released to the media.

## Codes of ethics

As technology advances and impacts the practice of nursing, a series of ethical concerns are raised. Professions address ethical concerns related to their duties and obligations through codes or guidelines. Codes of ethics for nursing provide a non-negotiable standard of care that details the ethical duties and obligations of every professional nurse. Codes of ethics express the profession's understanding of its commitment to society and to every individual in society. Since the earliest accounts of organised nursing, the Nightingale Pledge provided nurses with expectations for professional practice. It reads:

> I solemnly pledge myself before God and in the presence of this assembly, to pass my life in purity and to practice my profession faithfully. I will abstain from whatever is deleterious and mischievous, and will not take or knowingly administer any harmful drug. I will do all in my power to maintain and elevate the standard of my profession, and *will hold in confidence all personal matters committed to my keeping and all family affairs coming to my knowledge in the practice of my calling.* With loyalty will I endeavor to aid the physician in his work, and devote myself to the welfare of those committed to my care. (http://www.nursingworld.org/pressrel/nnw/printpledge.htm) (italics added)

This pledge was written at a time when the nature of communication was limited to direct conversations between persons or had written documents. As the italicised portion of the pledge states, the nurse was directly accountable for any breaches of confidential information, which holds true today. Disclosing any information in such a way that breaks patient confidentiality violates the spirit of the pledge.

The American Nurses Association (ANA) Code of Ethics for Nurses (ANA, 2001), hereafter referred to as the Code, addresses the need to maintain confidentiality of all patient information. The third provision of the Code states 'The nurse promotes, advocates for, and strives to protect the health, safety, and rights of the patient' (ANA, 2001, p. 12). Further explanation of this provision emphasises the duty to maintain confidentiality:

> Associated with the right to privacy, *the nurse has a duty to maintain confidentiality* of all patient information. The patient's well-being could be jeopardized and the fundamental trust between patient and the nurse destroyed by unnecessary access to data or by the inappropriate disclosure of identifiable patient information. The rights, well-being, and safety of the individual patient should be the primary factors in arriving at any professional judgment concerning the disposition of confidential information received from or about the patient, whether oral, written or *electronic*. The standard of nursing practice and the nurse's responsibility to provide quality care require that relevant data be shared with those members of the health care team who have a need to know. Only information pertinent to a patient's treatment and welfare is disclosed, and only to those directly involved with the patient's care. *Duties of confidentiality*, however, are not absolute and may need to be modified in order to protect the patient, other innocent parties, and in circumstances of mandatory disclosure for public health reasons. (p. 12)

The International Council of Nurses (ICN) has published a position statement, entitled *Health Information: Protection of Patient Rights*, which also addresses the issue of confidentiality of patient information (ICN, 2000). The ICN maintains that 'nurses must understand the ethical values and legal implications underlying their own responsibilities in respect for patients' right to privacy'. In its statement, the ICN recognises that health information systems pose threats to patients' right to privacy because of the increased accessibility of personal information. The ICN position statement supports national and international protocols for portable health records and supports the patient as the primary owner of their health information

### Breaches in confidentiality

As the distance between the onset and ending of any journey increases, the potential for unplanned events increases. Thus, it could be hypothesised that the greater the distance created by technology between the patient and the nurse, the greater the opportunity for an unplanned event, such as a breach of confidentiality. This is based on the belief that the most private and confidential exchange of information or communication occurs when it is exchanged between the shortest distance or face to face.

Breaches in confidentiality have always been a concern in health care. Intellectually, we are able to differentiate between discussions of patient information that are essential for the provision of care versus those that occur while socialising with other health professionals. However, there is evidence to support that health professionals do not always adhere to this duty Health professionals have been found to breach patient confidentiality when they talk about a patient while in an elevator with non-health care professionals at work or while in the midst of others in a public place (Ubel, et al., 1995, Vigod, Bell & Bohnen, 2003). A breach in patient confidentiality potentially occurs when messages are left on answering machines, when messages are left for persons for whom they were not intended. For example, leaving a message from a clinic could be a breach if other persons with access to the message system do not know about the clinic visit. These examples involve the potential of an uninvolved third party, who does not have an ethical responsibility to maintain privacy of patient information, to use this information, resulting in potentially harmful consequences.

When information is exchanged via e-mail or fax, there is also the potential for someone to see the written communication. Electronic mail creates both the lowest and highest potential for miscommunication of protected health information. On a lower level, the harm created by sending an e-mail message regarding the scheduling of an appointment that is subsequently read by another person is generally minimal. Additionally, unlike regular mail that may be delivered to an address that no longer belongs to a patient, an electronic mail message sent to the wrong address is almost always returned to the sender. Each e-mail address is unique to the individual, insofar as computerised servers do not allow duplication of addresses. On a higher level, there remains the potential for a greater breach of confidentiality, as is the case when an e-mail with extremely sensitive information is erroneously transmitted to a group of people or organisations listed on a distribution list. Distribution lists are lists of several different recipients under one group name. One slip of a mouse cursor on a list of contacts and an unintended group name could be inserted into the 'To': space. This situation occurred when a Health Department transmitted a list of HIV/AIDS patients to a group of community agencies for whom the information was not intended. In this case, personal information regarding this extremely private diagnosis was distributed to others who had no need to have this information. The ethical and legal consequences of a situation such as this are enormous.

Facsimiles (Faxes) carry a similar, but even greater potential for breach of privacy of patient information. One wrong digit on a fax number may result in personal information being sent to someone for whom this information is not intended. To illustrate, a chest X-ray result was faxed to an automobile dealer instead of the patient. This occurred in a small community where most people knew one another, and the X-ray finding of a lung tumour was now common knowledge of non-health professionals.

Distance technology is being used to provide consultation between a provider and a patient at a remote location. In certain instances, a patient may be in one location and the health professional in another location, possibly hundreds of miles away. The value of such service is great, particularly for individuals who are such a great distance from the health professional's location that the time and expense for commuting to the provider are prohibitive. While health information can be encrypted, there is still the potential for a transmission to be intercepted and information used for purposes other than for which it is intended. An additional concern with this type of interaction between patient and health professional is that without a relationship that is built on mutual trust and authentic presence, the quality and quantity of information being transmitted might be limited. The full benefit of a face-to-face consultation is therefore unachievable. Some clinics avoid this problem by requiring an initial face appointment before subsequent technology-mediated appointments.

## Trust

Trust is a fundamental component of the interaction between the patient and the nurse. In order to engage in the health care encounter, patients need to trust that the nurse will protect their health and safety, and the nurse needs to trust that patients will be honest and forthcoming about their pertinent personal information. Trust can be difficult to sustain in a virtual environment, wherein the patient and nurse may not have the opportunity to see one another face to face. When using a technological interface, the issue of maintaining confidentiality of information exchanged during the interaction is of utmost importance.

## 4.3 Protection of patient information – Legal implications

It is difficult to address ethics without also addressing law, in that laws generally follow events that conflict with societal norms and values. For example, laws about patient autonomy were promulgated in the United States following ethics cases where patients' wishes were not clear. The Patient Self Determination Act, passed in 1990, requires that all patients admitted to health care facilities receiving certain types of federal funding be given information about their rights regarding advance directives, to accept or refuse specific treatments and to direct their own health care decisions. Institutions are also required to document whether advance directives have been prepared and to provide education to community members regarding advance directives.

### Breach of confidentiality

While ethical practice is of great importance for patients and nurses, it is the legal recourse that essentially provides the consequences of any breach of confidential information. The ICN (2000) position statement, *Health Information: Protection of Patient Rights*, concludes with the sentence, 'Where this [patients right to privacy] is covered by the law, and nurses neglect their responsibilities under the law, they may have legal consequences.'

A breach of confidentiality of patient health information, regardless of the country in which it occurs, frequently involves legal consequences. In the United States, the consequences are addressed in federal legislation. The Health Insurance Portability and Accountability Act (HIPAA) is federal legislation that addresses the legal standards and consequences for not upholding patients' rights to protection of personal information (Code of Federal Regulations, 2002). The Act was primarily designed to minimise barriers to health insurance coverage, but with the increased exchange of information electronically, protection of this information was included in the law.

With advances in technology resulting in the electronic transmission of protected health information, concerns regarding the potential to intercept this information for uses other than patient care arose. Thus, regulations were added to HIPAA legislation and standards for privacy of personal health information were created. Failure to comply with HIPAA regulations could have civil and criminal penalties. The severity of the penalties increases according to the nature of the breach of confidentiality. Breaches that were unintended carry the lowest penalties, from $100 to $25,000 per year, and disclosure of private health information with the intent to sell for personal gain can result in penalties up to $250,000 and 10 years in prison (Frank-Stromberg, 2003). Legal implications of breaches of confidentially will vary among various countries around the world insofar as their laws frequently result from situations that challenge the basic values of the dominant philosophical, ethical and religious beliefs of societies.

### Duty to care and patient abandonment

Nurses and other health professionals have an ethical and legal obligation to attend to patients' needs. Legal liability for adverse outcomes that occur as a result of a professional relationship between a patient and a nurse results from an interaction in which this duty is either expressed or implied. When the nurse fails to respond to a patient in an appropriate amount of time, or unilaterally terminates any further interaction with the patient, patient abandonment results. The introduction of technology into the patient–nurse interaction creates new situations in which unintended claims of abandonment might potentially occur. The use of e-mail to initiate contact with a nurse or other health care professional is one example of a potential abandonment situation.

While there is no duty to respond to an unsolicited e-mail inquiry from a patient, once a response has taken place and provides or alludes to an assessment, diagnosis or recommendations being made, it would suggest that the health care provider had undertaken the provision of care. In this case, failure to respond appropriately puts the nurse at risk for accusation of abandonment. The exception to this is a case in which an emergency situation exists. Good samaritan legislation provides immunity for those health professionals who respond according to an appropriate standard of care.

Abandonment can occur unintentionally when technical difficulties arise. During a detailed or critical explanation of health information, decreased access to the Internet might occur. The provider needs to know if the information was received by the patient. Without an alternative plan for service delivery, the patient could potentially suffer an adverse event.

### Negligence and malpractice

Providing advice to patients over a phone has been recognised as potentially rife with danger. Knowledge of a particular patient is necessary for appropriate diagnosis and treatment. When vague or non-definitive symptoms are discussed with the health care provider by any mode of electronic communication, a risk of inaccurate diagnosis exists. Inevitably, a number of wrong decisions will be made or wrong advice given. Follow up and evaluation are possible using electronic communication, but clear plans for follow up need to be developed.

One situation where electronic communication had the potential to result in a serious outcome occurred when an e-mail arrived in a telehealth triage centre from a mother requesting information about a type of lozenges that could be used for her child's sore throat. A quick response to this request might have been to simply provide the name of a lozenge. However, the provider decided that a more thorough assessment of the situation was indicated. The provider was able to determine that the child was a toddler who was not yet able to communicate verbally but that he was drooling and not eating. Knowing that these were signs of possible epiglottitis, the provider instructed the mother to take the child to the emergency room. The child required intubation and mechanical ventilation soon thereafter. If the nurse had not taken the time to obtain more details about the situation, the child might not have survived. Nurses are accustomed to envisioning potential difficulties that patients might experience in the clinical setting. That imagination must be extended when using electronic media rather than face-to-face contact for patient care.

## 4.4  Tele-health nursing

Tele-health nursing covers a range of technologies that include telephone triage or call centres, two-way interactive video such as is used in home care and using high-tech equipment. In the United States, telehealth is defined as the use of electronic information and telecommunications technologies to support long-distance clinical health care, patient and professional health-related education, public health and health administration (Puskin & Kumekawa, 2001).

Tele-health nursing developed in the United States in response to the restructuring of the health care system to increase quality and access of care and to minimise cost (Hutcherson, 2001). Such technology, however, is not limited to the United States as telephone triage or call centres are present in other countries worldwide. This raises the possibility that the care provider for a particular patient could be actually operating from a country different from that of the patient. This has the possibility of providing care where it would otherwise not be accessible. On the other hand, misunderstanding and a lack of cultural awareness or sensitivity are possible.

Two-way interactive video encounters are increasingly being used to supplement home care services. It is now possible for home-bound patients to be assisted in drawing up and self-administering insulin with the guidance and feedback of a professional nurse at the other end of a video transmission. Patients with congestive heart failure can place an electronic stethoscope on their chest while the nurse can listen to the transmitted lung sounds to determine the presence of adventitious breath sounds. Web-based technology allows for the transmission of images of wounds. This extends the use of the technology from providing history or subjective data to providing objective data that is obtained at the direction of the distant care provider. The ability to increase access of home-bound individuals living in remote geographic areas to nursing care is phenomenal.

The missing component in these encounters is that a *hands-on* encounter has not taken place. It is this missing component that provides the basis for the challenge that telehealth nursing is not actual nursing practice, and therefore should not be regulated by nursing. However, boards of nursing have analysed the practice of telehealth nursing and have determined that it utilises the knowledge, judgement and critical thinking that is at the crux of nursing education and is indeed the practice of nursing (Hutcherson, 2001). To address the issue of standardisation of knowledge necessary for telehealth nursing, the American Academy for Ambulatory Nursing Care (AAANC), in conjunction with the Nurses Credentialing Center, has developed a certification process for telephone nursing practice, a component of telehealth nursing. Among the competencies required of registered nurses who are certified in telephone nursing practice are being able to use algorithms or protocols to support decision making, assess whether an actual or potential health, safety, or educational need exists, and develop a plan of care with their providers and support systems.

## 4.5 Ethical implications of telehealth nursing

### Justice

Telehealth nursing has the ability to both increase and decrease access to health care. It helps facilitate access of isolated and geographically remote persons to health information, thereby addressing nursing's commitment to distributive justice. By bringing health care to these areas, individuals do not need to travel long distances to see health care providers, thus saving both time and money. On the contrary, many areas of the country do not have the necessary structure to accommodate telecommunications and thereby have the potential to experience further disparities in the ability to access care.

Another benefit of bringing care to the patient is that patients become less reliant on health care facilities, which will have an additional effect on reducing costs (Coleman, 2002). In some small way, the ability of patients to be seen in their own home rather than travelling to a facility allows them to have more control over their days and thus increased autonomy. On the contrary, those persons living in areas without access to technology are further marginalised because they have no other alternative than to travel to a facility that is miles away from home, requiring transportation that is costly in terms of lost work as well as in direct cost of the transportation itself. Many of these facilities may no longer exist as telehealth supplants the physical structures for delivery of care.

### Beneficence

Beneficence is the ethical principles concerned with doing good. The benefits to patients' use of electronic technology in terms of cost and time savings have be discussed. There are additional benefits that can occur. Johnson-Mekota, et al. (2001) found that more than 55 per cent of patients participating in a telehealth nursing service identified their satisfaction as very high. Using the nursing process as the framework to study the quality of telehealth nursing, Chang, Mayo and Omery (2002) determined that there was a significant relationship between the quality of the intervention and patients' satisfaction. In their integrative review of eleven studies in which patients participated in a telehealth service with a video component, Thurmond and Boyle (2002) found that all of the patients and their caretakers were satisfied with the service. Other studies have shown that telehealth can decrease office visits, hospital days and intensive care days (Fisher, 1995).

## 4.6 Accessing health information electronically

Health information includes information for staying well, preventing and managing disease, and making decisions related to health and health care. Roy (2000) identified patients' computer access to health information as one of the major trends to shape the future of nursing care. The issue of Internet access to health information creates a multitude of ethical issues for nursing practice. While there are many reputable websites providing health information, there are also many other sites that promote questionable information and anecdotal or untested interventions. The issue of protecting patients from receiving incorrect information and inappropriate and untested interventions becomes a critical concern. Control of website development and content is minimal, which means that information that the website developers or owners include on the site may not be correct, or even worse, unsafe. As more and more patients use the Internet to learn about various diseases and conditions, it is important for nurses and other health care providers to have some level of understanding about what these websites include.

A well-developed website with reference to evidence may not meet the rigor of scientific evidence, and may be more convincing than the evidence that a health care provider may be able to provide during a brief patient encounter. To illustrate, a patient may be interested in using magnet therapy for the treatment of chronic back pain. Perhaps the patient has searched the Internet for information and has studied all of the sites and comes to the conclusion that magnet therapy is superior to the use of any other therapeutic modality. The nurse or other health care provider may have a very difficult time even getting the patient to listen to information regarding other types of treatment for chronic back pain. The ethical principle of respect for autonomy would result in the nurse not attempting to change the patient's decision; however, the lack of scientific evidence comparing this modality to other modalities with substantial scientific evidence might in turn suggest that the provider was not practicing beneficently in this situation. The balancing of respect for autonomy and benefi-cence becomes the critical ethical dilemma for the nurse. It would be important to leave the door open for the patient to return for care if they find that their chosen therapy is not effective. In other cases where patients might be consid-ering the refusal of proven treatment such as chemotherapy for breast cancer in preference for vitamins, nurses could openly communicate their thoughts about treatment effectiveness, but allow patients to reconsider their choices at a later time.

Enhancing the use of Internet-based health information may be viewed as enhancing patient autonomy. Instead of demanding that all health information be controlled and provided by the patient's providers, patients have the potential to search the web to obtain information. In the United States, the government regulates the content and postings of many health information sites. The Federal Trade Commission (FTC) regulates false and deceptive advertising. The Food and Drug Administration (FDA) regulates safe medical devices and products. Apart from governmental sponsored or approved Internet sites, a large number of proprietary or industry-sponsored sites exist. Essentially, almost anyone can have a website with health information. Many times, developers of these sites have the potential of financial gain, if they are promoting and/or selling their own miracle drugs or interventions. The potential for financial gain raises concern over whether the suggestions are being made for therapeutic versus monetary gain. Without some type of accreditation or approval mechanism for the sites, the only way to discern the site's credibility is to follow up with a review of the scientific literature for evidence to support the intervention.

## Self-directed health education

Patient education has historically been provided face to face with patients. Education about disease processes and how to prevent or manage them has been part of the traditional health care encounter. Over the years, other forms of health education technologies have been instituted. Initially, this included printed materials to supplant verbal instructions and eventually the use of films, audiotapes and videotapes. More recent technologies include interactive software, in which the patient interacts with a computer program for the purpose of engaging in a decision-making process which provides immediate feedback for incorrect and correct responses. With the rapid emergence of the Internet and subsequent health-related websites, a wide variety of informational and educational materials are available to anyone having access to a computer.

The positive aspect of this accessibility to information is that patients have the freedom to explore their health concerns in their own timeframe, rather than that of the provider. Since many chronic disease processes require a change in behaviour, such as a change in nutritional intake or implementation of a medication regimen, the delivery of this information needs to be according to patients' readiness to change. Behaviour change theory emphasises that change is very individualised. Historically, patient education to change a behaviour occurred at the convenience of the provider, typically during a hospitalisation or at the time of discharge. However, determining individual patient learning styles, assessing existing knowledge and tailoring educational plans to accommodate patient needs is a very timely process. Through the development of computerised educational programs, patients can enter personal data, existing knowledge of their disease and condition and preferred learning styles, and subsequently an individualised program of instruction is automatically created. Many of these computerised self-directed programs can be completed over a period of time, allowing the patient to control the amount of information obtained in their preferred timeframe. Programs that assess the individual needs of patients and tailor the education to meet those needs represent respect for the individual patient's autonomy.

While all of this sounds ideal, this is not always the case. The Internet is a publicly accessible means of providing information. The control of what can be entered on the Internet is intentionally not rigid, in order to allow the free flow of communication internationally. Unfortunately, incorrect information may also be accessible. To potentially undiscerning patients, this information could result in significant harm and possibly even death.

In order to prevent the distribution of potentially harmful information, oftentimes made available by well-intended individuals, several safeguards have been implemented. Several health-related organisations have developed guidelines for Internet sites that provide health and medical information. One of the most credible sources of information is that which is posted on government sites. Governments are entrusted to provide safe environments for citizens, exemplified in the broadest of examples by departments of defence. Just as citizens need to be safe from larger threats of war or environmental issues, they need to be protected from unregulated health information.

In addition to governmental safeguards put forth through regulatory policies and procedures, non-governmental agencies have come forth to address the issue of the safety of health information on the Internet. Health on the Net (HON) is a non-profit international agency with the sole purpose of reviewing Internet sites and determining the accuracy and appropriateness of the health information they are providing. Sites that meet rigorous standards receive a HON stamp of approval, which allows them to include a HON icon on their home page.

The HON organisation, based in Switzerland, was developed in 1996 and addressed the reliability and credibility of content on health web sites.

Several other health-related organisations have developed guidelines for Internet sites that provide health and medical information (Table 4.1).

Guidelines, logos and certifications have been established to demonstrate upholding of certain principles. Consumer-oriented sites have also been developed and provide actual ratings or checklists for evaluating the health-related websites (see Table 4.2). Patients can be referred to the approved sites for health-related information.

Although governmental sites and HON make strides towards the protection of patients, even the most correct information accessed at a potentially inappropriate time can cause considerable harm. This is where the role of health professionals such as nurses can take the lead in assessing the emotional readiness and support that might be necessary for patients to learn about particular aspects of the disease, condition or treatment. An example of how this might be harmful is that an individual who has not established a relationship with a health care provider might attend a community health screening and learn that he/she has high cholesterol. The individual might return home and conduct a computer

**Table 4.1**  Health and medical Internet site evaluation

| Organisation | Logo | Guidelines | Website address | Certification process | Ethical code of conduct |
|---|---|---|---|---|---|
| American Medical Association | | X | http://jama.ama-assn.org/cgi/ content/full/283/12/1600 | | |
| Health on the Net | HONcode | X | http://www.hon.ch/ HONcode | X | |
| Health Internet Ethics (Hi-Ethics) | | X | http://www.hiethics.org/ Principles/index.asp | | X |
| Internet Health care Coalition (IHC) | | X | http://www.ihealthcoalition. org/ethics/ethics.html | | X |
| National Association of Boards of Pharmacy | VIPPS | X | http://www.nabp.net/ | X | |
| TRUSTe | TRUSTe | X | www.truste.org | | |

**Table 4.2**  Consumer Internet site evaluation

| Website | Address | Rating mechanism |
|---|---|---|
| Health on the Net (HON) | http://www.hon.ch/HONcode/ HONcode_check.html | Consumer evaluates with HONcode site-checker. |
| Internet Health care Coalition | http://www.ihealthcoalition.org/ content/tips.html | Ten suggestions for consumer evaluation of sites. |
| University of Oxford, Division of Public Health and Primary Health Care | http://www.discern.org.uk | DISCERN questionnaire. Consumer evaluates written information about treatment choices. |

search and find out a number of unproven remedies to control cholesterol. Not knowing the difference between scientific evidence for interventions and poten-tially fictitious information (provided by someone who has the ability to profit monetarily from their purported cures) may lead to delayed treatment and pos-sible bad outcomes. One approach that a health care provide can take is to ask the patient to bring in or forward the sites they are considering so that the provider can correct potential errors or help to determine appropriateness for the particular patient. This is potentially very time-consuming, but can support other patient education activities.

There are many ethical implications of increasing accessibility to health infor-mation. The first is that respect for autonomy would lead the health care provider to the conclusion that individuals should have the freedom and right to access information and to make their own decisions. The principle of beneficence frequently provides an alternate view to autonomy. It is this balancing of respect for autonomy and beneficence which consumes much of the ethical decision making in health care. As a health care provider, upholding the principle of beneficence by assisting a patient in the selection of health information is of utmost importance. The principle of non-maleficence would guide the health care provider to be concerned that no harm would result from the patient's self-directed search for information and subsequent self-treatment. The principle of justice provides an interesting perspective on the availability of information on the Internet.

The assumption that access to health information on the net is available to everyone is short-sighted. This view is based on the belief that all patients have equal access to the Internet and that information is available to all people, regardless of their language. As more and more patients are directed to the Internet as standard practice to obtain health information, there is the potential to inadvertently exclude entire populations (Maddox, 2002). This situation challenges the ethical principle of justice and has the potential of creating a second-tiered system of care. For those who believe that the use of electronic modalities to access and transmit health information is essential for the improvement of public health, the provision of low-cost or loaned computers to the needy, with discounted access to online services, is believed to be a mechanism for increasing health knowledge and reducing health disparities (Eng & Gustafson, 1999).

The issue of personal choice is raised as Internet communication technologies permeate our health care system. How much choice do patients have when choosing their preferred mode of communication? While computer availability and Internet access can be easily provided, the issue of patient choice is more difficult to address. If a health care provider decides that all messages need to be sent electronically, rather than by phone (assuming everyone has Internet access), how much choice might an individual patient have to opt out of this mode of communication? There might be a certain amount of justification for using electronic communication for documentation of messages, insofar as information written by the patient would be entered into the permanent health record rather than left verbally on a voice message, wherein there is the potential for misunderstanding due to different levels of health literacy. However, if respect for persons is upheld, then respect for their desired mode of communication should follow.

Communication via e-mail might sound logically appealing, but there is little evidence to support this and many other electronic health services. Maddox (2002) challenges whether ethical principles have been used to guide the decision to use unproven electronic health technologies. She questions whether it is the utilitarian perspective of the 'greater good' which has lead to the endorsement of technologies that have been proven neither to be cost-effective nor efficient.

## 4.7 Strategies for upholding ethical practice in nursing

Because of the concerns about privacy and accuracy of health information exchange, leaders in the area of telehealth recognised the need for standards or guidelines for its use. Individual agencies or organisations have begun to implement standards, but for a more global approach to standardisation, the Internet Healthcare Coalition established the eHealth Code of Ethics (Rippen & Risk, 2000). This code was established in order to ensure that persons have a full understanding of the risks and benefits of using the Internet in managing their own and others' health care. The principal goal of the code is to help create a trustworthy environment for all health care users: patients, nurses, other health care professionals and website sponsors.

The eHealth Code of Ethics (Rippen & Risk, 2000) identifies several guiding principles for creating ethically justifiable use of Internet technology. These values include candour, honesty, quality of information, products and services, informed consent, privacy, professionalism, responsible partnering and accountability. Respect for persons is the principle philosophical foundation of the eHealth of Ethics. This principle is also the fundamental provision within the ANA Code of Ethics for Nurses. Individual nurses must be vigilant as technology is introduced into the practice arena. Determining whether patient privacy is protected in all the potential ways that information can now be transmitted may require that nurses sit on information technology committees in their health care setting. On the other hand, while protecting patient privacy, we must not isolate the patient as care is delivered. For example, the goal for patients in acute care may be to return to the home setting. Communicating about home transition and care will require communicating with more than just the patient. At every level, the nurse must exert judgements about appropriate types and levels of communication as well as appropriate audiences and participants in care. Technology-mediated communication increases the demand on nursing judgement.

The importance of maintaining protection of patient information, and of patient confidentiality, is a critical element of the ethical utilisation of technology in nursing. Privacy rules established by the HIPAA act address the transmission of protected health information over the Internet, Extranet, phone lines, or information that is moved from one location to another using magnetic tape (audiotapes dictation or patient encounters) or computer disks. Health-related transactions, such as requests for payment from insurance companies and request for health records from one provider to another, are also covered by this privacy rule. Communicating information necessary for care delivery is not barred by HIPAA rules.

Rules created by laws that restrict the transmission or transaction of health information have the potential of interfering with the timeliness of referrals to other health care providers and sharing of health information for the purpose of setting up appointments or consultations. These activities fit the definition of treatment under the privacy rule. Unlike the laws enacted to address protection of patient information, codes of ethics are voluntary standards that serve to set out the importance of certain activities or behaviours, educate persons involved with the practice governed by the code and identify the values that shape best practices (Crigger, 2002).

### Recommendations for influencing health policy

One of the requirements having the greatest impact on health care providers is that all employees requiring access to protected patient information must be trained in the regulations regarding protection of information (Frank-Stromberg, 2003). Policies and procedures regarding the training of employees and protection of information must be in place in every institution. Health care providers cannot hide behind information privacy laws and fail to communicate essential patient information. When HIPAA was first enacted, rumours were spread that nurses were not allowed to discuss patient conditions even with family members. Realising that patients might choose to communicate with some, but no all, family members requires a full nursing assessment. Who are the patient's preferences for support? This information must be made clear in patient records so that the health care team can provide appropriate care.

It is essential to assure that nurses engage in the practice of telehealth nursing and curricula development for increasing knowledge so that the ethical implications are clearly addressed. The American Academy of Ambulatory Care Nursing (AAACN) developed a Tele-health Nursing Practice Core Course (TNPCC) to address the essential components for the practice of telehealth nursing. This or similar courses which include the ethical implications of tele-health technology need to be incorporated into nursing curricula.

eHealth is still a consumer-beware environment which requires a certain level of sophistication to be able to negotiate the Internet and evaluate the quality of health information. The Internet is a powerful tool which has the potential to improve health by enhancing the care received. On the other hand, if not used wisely and discretely, it can create some of the most horrendous situations. Nurses as patient advocates must be part of policy development and implementation for emerging eHealth technologies. If nurses regularly ask patients what their sources of health-related information is when establishing the nursing assessment, they can use this information to provide essential guidance for patients in identifying high-quality information sources.

### 4.8 Final reflection

The need for nurses to uphold the ethical practice of nursing while engaging in technologies that impact the patient–nurse interaction has been the focus of this chapter. Electronic communication and accessing health information via the Internet have had the greatest impact on this interaction. Nursing is a communication-based profession. Technology that enhances or substitutes for face-to-face communication is thus of ultimate concern. Technological advances have the potential to lure patients and health care providers into the belief that technology is concomitant with state-of-the-art health care. Those who support this view have the potential for dehumanising the environments in which technology is used. The lure of precision, standardisation, objectivity and efficiency create the potential of losing sight on the uniqueness of each patient.

Nurses must not lose sight of the need to focus on caring for the patient and his/her experience of being ill. As our culture increasingly focuses on technology as the solution to most human problems, the nurse must 'uphold the overall well being of the patient and advocate for the patient, not the technology' (Drought & Liaschenko, 1995, p. 304).

What the future holds is up to nurses. Nurses must not fight the rising tide of technology, nor must they float passively along. The ability for nurses to advocate for patients will enhance the ability for positive outcomes to occur. Nursing has the responsibility to become involved in developing the guidelines, regulations and processes that will facilitate tele-health nursing, while maintaining a keen focus on not diminishing the appreciation of caring skills. Nurses must conduct research that addresses the meaning of technology and caring. Technology's goodness or badness is related to its use. As long as the patient remains nursing's primary focus, technology will be just another instrument.

John Naisbett, the author of *Megatrends*, most aptly summarised the placement of technology in our lives; he stated: 'We must learn to balance the material wonders of technology with the spiritual demands of our human nature. In our wonderful technological world let us also celebrate our humanness' (Naisbett, 2002).

## LEARNING ACTIVITIES

1. Identify one website directed to consumers of health care. Evaluate the quality of information as regards currency, readability and usefulness from the consumer's perspective.

2. Go to the website of the nursing association for your country. Determine whether there is a policy addressing the role of the nurse with respect to communications technology. What should an appropriate policy stress?

3. In small groups identify one potential ethical dilemma related to the use of information technology from a practice area. Why is there a problem and what are the key issues?

4. Survey a group of consumers regarding their use and perception of health-related information. Would they prefer to speak directly to a health care provider regarding their health concerns, or would they prefer to investigate health information using information technology on their own? Are there specific issues they would prefer to search anonymously?

## References

American Nurses Association. (2001). *Code of Ethics for Nurses with Interpretive Statements.* Washington, DC: American Nurses Publishing.

Barnard, A. (1997). A critical review of the belief that technology is a neutral object and nurses are its master. *Journal of Advanced Nursing, 26,* 126–131.

Barnard, A. (2000). Alteration to will is an experience of technology and nursing. *Journal of Advanced Nursing, 31,* 1136–1144.

Beidler, S. M. (2002). Ethical issues experienced by primary care nurse practitioners caring for vulnerable patients in nursing centers. *Dissertation Abstracts International, 63*(5), 2300B. (UMI No. 3054922).

Chang, B. L., Mayo, A. & Omery, A. (2002). Evaluating quality of telehealth advice nursing. *Western Journal of Nursing Research, 24,* 583–590.

Code of Federal Regulations. (2002). *45 CFR parts 160 and 164. Standards for Privacy of Individual Identifiable Health Information.* [Retrieved 31 July 2005] http://www.hhs.gov. ezproxy.fau.edu/ocr/hippa/privacy.html

Coleman, J. R. (2002). MCO Trends: HMOs and the future of telemedicine. *Case Manager, 13*(4), 38–43.

Crigger, B. (2002). *Foundations of the eHealth Code of Ethics. Internet Healthcare Coalition.* [Retrieved 31 August 2005] from http://www.ihealthcoalition.org/ethics/code-foundations.html.

Drought, T. S. & Liaschenko, J. (1995). Ethical practice in a technological age. *Critical Care Nursing Clinics of North America, 7*(2), 297–304.

Eng, T. R. & Gustafson, D. (1999). *Wired for Health and Well-being: The Emergence of Interactive Health Communication.* Washington, DC: US Government Printing Office.

Fisher, G. R. (1995). Telemedicine and the payment system. *Pennsylvania Medicine, 98*(11), 32–34.

Frank-Stromberg, M. (2003). They're real and they're here: The new federally regulated privacy rules under HIPAA. *MEDSURG Nursing, 12*(6), 380–385, 414.

Gallagher, S. M. (2000). Ethics: The ethics of advanced technology. *Ostomy/wound Management, 46*(8), 10, 12, 14. (8 ref 5 bb).

Hagerty, B. M. & Patusky, K. L. (2003). Reconceptualizing the nurse-patient relationship. *Journal of Nursing Scholarship, 35*(2), 145–150.

Hutcherson, C. M. (2001). Legal considerations for nurses practicing in a telehealth setting. *Online Journal of Issues in Nursing, 6*(3), 10.

International Council of Nurses (ICN). (2000). *Health Information: Protection of Patient Rights.* [Retrieved 15 September 2005] http://www.icn.ch/pspatinetsrights00.htm.

Johnson-Mekota, J. L., Maas, M., Buresh, K. A., Gardner, S. E., Frantz, R. A., & Specht, J. K. P. et al. (2001). A nursing application of telecommunications: Measurement of satisfaction for patients and providers. *Journal of Gerontological Nursing, 27*(1), 28–33.

King, I. M. (1981). *Toward a Theory for Nursing.* New York: John Wiley.

Maddox, P. J. (2002). Ethics and the brave new world of e-health. *Online Journal of Nursing Issues,* [Retrieved 19 February 2004] http://www.nursingworld.org/ojin/ethicol/ethics_10.htm.

Meleis, A. I. (1997). *Theoretical Nursing: Development and Progress* (3rd edn.). Philadelphia, PA: Lippincott.

Morse, J. M. (1991). Negotiating commitment and involvement in the nurse-patient relationship. *Journal of Advanced Nursing, 16,* 455–468.

Naisbett, J. (2002). High tech, high touch: John Naisbett's world view. *Caring, 21*(4), 24–27.

Peplau, H. E. (1987). Interpersonal constructs for nursing practice. *Nurse Education Today, 7*(5), 201–208.

Peplau, H. E. (1992). Interpersonal relations: A theoretical framework for application in nursing practice. *Nursing Science Quarterly, 5*(1), 13–18.

Puskin, D. & Kumekawa, J. (2001). *2001 Telemedicine Report to Congress.* Rockville, MD: Department of Health and Human Services, Health Resources and Services Administration, Office for the Advancement of Technology.

Rippen, H. & Risk, A. (2000). e-Health Code of Ethics. *Journal of Medical Internet Research, 2*(2), Article e9. [Retrieved 31 August 2005] http://www.jmir.org/2000/2/e9/index.htm

Roy, C. (2000). The visible and invisible fields that shape the future of the nursing care system. *Nursing Administration Quarterly, 25*(1), 119–131.

Thurmond, V. A. & Boyle, D. K. (2002). An integrative review of patients' perceptions regarding telehealth used in their health care. *Online Journal of Knowledge Synthesis for Nursing, 9*(2), Document Number 2, 21.

Ubel, P. A., Zell, M. M., Miller, D. J., Fischer. G. S., Peters-Stefani, D. & Arnold, R. M. (1995). Elevator talk: Observational study of inappropriate comments in a public space. *American Journal of Medicine, 99*, 190–194.

Vigod, S. N., Bell, C. M. & Bohnen, J. M. A. (2003). Privacy of patients' information in hospital lifts: Observational study. *British Medical Journal, 327*(7422), 1024–1025.

---

### RECOMMENDED READING

Crigger, B. J. (2001). Foundations of the ehealth code of ethics. *Internet Healthcare Coalition.* www.ihealthcoalition.org/ethics/ehealthcode0524.html

Maddox, P. J. (2002). Ethics and the brave new world of e-health. *Online Journal of Issues in Nursing.* www.nursingworld.org/ojin/ethicol/ethics_10.htm

Thurmond, V. A. & Boyle, D. K. (2002). An integrative review of patients' perceptions regarding tele-health used in their health care. *The Online Journal of Knowledge Synthesis for Nursing, 9* (Document number 2).

# Paediatric Community Nursing: The Experience of Caring for Technology-Dependent Children at Home

Katherine Wang, Alan Barnard and
Margarette Somerville

## LEARNING OBJECTIVES

When you have read this chapter, you will be able to:

- Explain the changes as the result of introducing medical technology into a home.

- Discuss the challenges for community nurses with paediatric home care.

- Identify key issues for care of a child depending on medical technology at home.

- Discuss the care-giving experiences and needs of families of in-home technology-dependent children.

## KEY WORDS

- care

- carers

- community nursing

- family

- home

- paediatric nursing

- technology

- technology-dependent children

## 5.1 Introduction

If we are to consider community nursing for children and medical technology together, then perhaps it may lead to rather unsettling thoughts because the two do not usually come to mind harmoniously. Home care, particularly for children, often means family, privacy, comfort and safety (Edgü & Ünlü, 2003; Reed, 1996). However, when care is subject to the use of medical equipment or the constant presence of an outside carer in the home, it can become the centre of attention and changes occur to the meaning of relationships. For example, the relationships between parent and child, child and carer, parent and carer or family and home may carry different meanings that are not made clear in current literature. As the result of a lack of evidence, families of in-home technology-dependent children have been receiving insufficient and inappropriate support, and can experience stress and burden of care to a level harmful to their health (Heaton, et al., 2005; Miles, et al., 1999; Ratliffe, et al., 2002; Stephenson, 1999; Thyen, Kuhlthau & Perrin, 1999; Wang, 2005).

There is urgent need to understand the meaning and impacts of 'technology' within the home of a technology-dependent child. This chapter provides an overview of the experiences of a group of carers (i.e. parents and nurses/carers) who care for a child depending on medical and technical care at home. Discussion of care issues in relation to medical care and machinery will be presented along with examples that draw on the words of parents or nurses/carers who care for technology-dependent children in the community (Wang, 2005). The chapter is presented in two parts however both draw on the perspectives of parents and nurses/carers caring for a technology-dependent child at home. The first part presents and discusses care in relation to the meaning of discharging a technology-dependent child to home and the impact of medical care and machinery on the lives of individuals in the home. The second part discusses issues of psychological and social care of children and families living with medical technology at home.

## 5.2 The experience of caring for technology-dependent children at home: An Australian experience

A qualitative study was undertaken from 2001 to 2005 that included interviews with seventeen primary caregivers who cared for a child with a tracheostomy dependent upon intermittent or continuous respiratory support at home (Wang, 2005). The caregivers were recruited from four different health care institutions across four states of Australia. After ethics approval participants were contacted and informed about the research via telephone and both oral and written consents were gained prior to face-to-face interviews. The research approach of phenomenography was chosen for data collection, analysis and interpretation (Barnard, McCosker & Gerber, 1999; Marton, 1981, 1986, 1988, 2000; Marton & Booth, 1997). Interviews were conducted in homes and their length ranged from 45–90 minutes. Interviews were taped recorded and transcribed verbatim and quotations from participants that appear in this chapter have been provided with pseudonyms. Open-ended questions included in the interviews included for example, 'What does caring for your child at home mean for you?' or 'What is a typical day for you?' A seven phase analysis was undertaken (Dahlgren & Fallsberg, 1991), and Atlas.ti, a qualitative data analysis software was used to assist data organisation.

Research findings included seven categories of description and an outcome space (a diagram depicting the phenomenon under investigation) (Wang, 2005). The care-giving experiences of the primary caregivers are described as 'Hospital is another world to me' (1), 'It's a new world' (2), an ambiguous social identity (3), 'The medical technology associated with my child is frightening but necessary' (4), 'The difficulty is having the carers at home' (5), social isolation (6) and the experience as changing as a person (7). The seven categories of description relate to each other in a specific way in terms of meaning and structure, and together were represented diagrammatically as an outcome space which described an understanding of the 'new world' of the primary caregiver caring for a ventilator-dependent child at home.

### Care at home

Parents and lay carers must undertake some level of medical training while in hospital prior to taking a technology-dependent child home (Figure 5.1). For instance, one mother explained that:

> they showed us how to use all the different machines that we have … a ventilator, a heart and oxygen monitor, and one of these face mask pumps for breathing. So they gave us a couple of hours training in each of those … gave us a refresher on CPR. It was really only a couple of hours over a couple of days.

Discharging a child home dependent on medical and technical care requires not only training of parents and carers but also the appropriate organisation of funding for initial and ongoing needs of the child and family. Accessing funding for home care for technology-dependent children can be a challenge because eligibility for funding is too often limited. As of 2004 in Queensland, Australia, to receive government funding for assistance to care for a ventilator-dependent child, the child must require invasive ventilation for 24 h per day (criteria varied slightly across different states of Australia at the time). The criteria means children who are medically stable yet partially dependent on ventilation assistance can experience insufficient funding for home care. Appropriate financial assistance is crucial to the successful discharge of a technology-dependent child and is equally essential for the maintenance of quality care and life for the child and

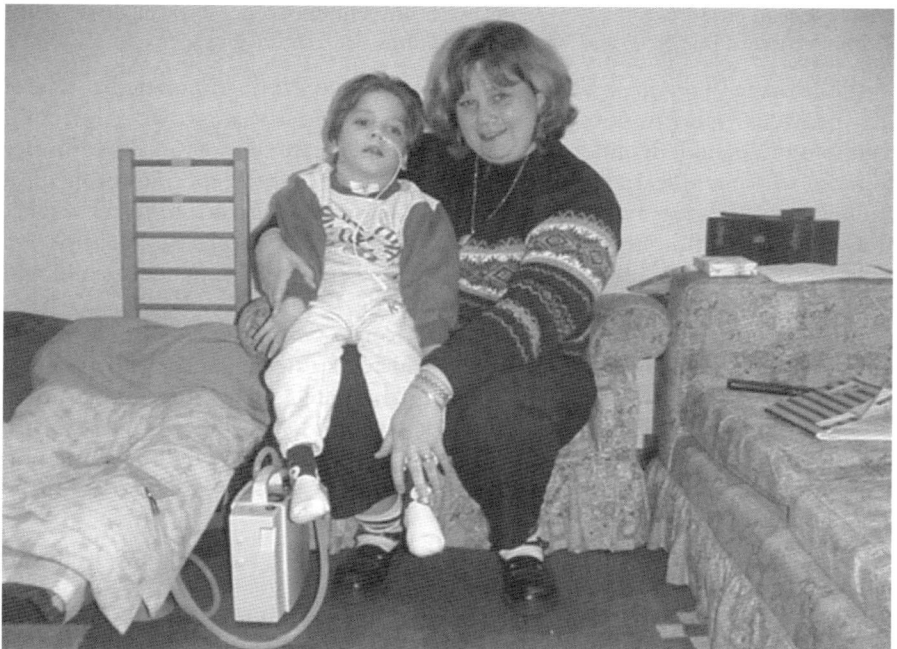

**Figure 5.1**   A child and mother at home together.

their family. For example, a mother of a seven-year-old boy with a tracheostomy needing 24 hour's ventilation support revealed that

> We've been very lucky because most of ours has been provided by the Health Department ... I don't know how we would have coped ... because, the medical costs of what he has to have since he's been home would be phenomenal ... We probably wouldn't have been able to do it, and he'd be still in hospital.

Although funding is always in shortage, it is necessary for the success of caring for technology-dependent children at home. Progress in physical growth and motor skills of the child is often the first sign of the success of home care, and similarly the stimulation of a home environment can be important for a child. For example, a boy with a Congenital Central Hypoventilation Syndrome (CCHS – a disorder of the central nervous system where the automatic control of breathing is impaired or absent that result in hypoxia or hypercapnia) was not home until he was four years old:

> He learnt sign language but as soon as we got home he stopped and started talking. He knew there was a drink in the fridge; he never knew what a fridge was before that. He knew there was biscuits in the cupboard or, knew how to turn the telly on or stereo ... . Like, the first time he flushed the toilet he started dancing to it, he thought it was music ... and then the first time I had a shower he started crying because he'd never seen me with no clothes on and he was frightened by all the water coming on me in this box ... We'd put him into bed with us and he didn't know what

to do, just sitting like this you know, what am I meant to do? I mean there're just hundreds and hundreds and hundreds of things you can imagine.

While home nurtures the children with safety and stimulations, school also provides opportunities for developmental and social growth. Enabling technology-dependent children to attend school creates opportunities for other children to see and learn about their specific needs and the specifics of medical equipment. It is a learning opportunity for others and a chance to foster respect and acceptance of difference. School is a primary place where the identity of a child is formed. The same is true both for the technology-dependent child and sibling(s) who may often go to the same school.

Although caring for a child depending on technical care at home brings positive outcomes for the child, it will lead to stress and burden for families who are living with the child. The daily instrumental care of the child at home is demanding and stressful. For example, one single mother who cares for a seventeen-years-old child with a tracheostomy who depends on 24 h ventilation assistance described her responsibility to provide medical care everyday in the following way:

> A typical day is we have carers go at seven so I get up at half past six ... and have coffee and do the school lunches for Peter (the younger sibling) and then get Peter's school things ready and then I go into Daniel (the ventilator-dependent child) then the carer goes. I get Daniel up from bed, he goes into the lounge and lays on a type of bed which goes up and down. He lays on there, I do his catheterisation for his urine ... and then he has breakfast, Ozmolite milk ... with the gastrostomy and medicines. Then, at half past seven I wake Peter up to get ready for school ... Peter and I have breakfast. And then Peter goes to school and so I get Daniel dressed. Get Peter sorted out and ... he catches the bus out the front. Then, I start with Daniel. I can give Daniel a shower and ... he's got a pressure sore which I do a dressing on it ... a pressure sore on the top of his leg which he's had for five years ... they say will never heal because to heal it's got to be off it for six to eight weeks ... but he can't be totally off it because then the ventilator doesn't ventilate the lungs properly and he ends up with a chest infection. So we've sort of got to manage it up and down. At ten o'clock, the access cab comes and picks Daniel up with the registered nurse and takes him to school. When he goes to school, I do the household chores ... Daniel gets home at four o'clock in the access cab and I make sure I'm always home by then if I go out ... I do his catheterisation when he first comes home. He has water as extra fluid through his gastrostomy tube. He likes to do some eating for about an hour usually. And then I get him down off his bottom for the pressure sore ... and he has Ozmolite milk for his tea ... and watches the telvision. I come out and cook tea. Peter and I have our tea ... give Daniel a bit of a wash. He has medicines and Ozmolite milk again for the fourth lot. At half past nine, I put him into bed and get all that sorted out, like with the ventilators and the suction cases ... the carer comes at ten o'clock and stays in the bedroom with him.

Mobilising a child needing numerous medical machines around a house is itself a challenge considering the way a conventional house in Australia is designed and built. For example, a family with a ventilator-dependent child confronted the task of trying to manoeuvre a wheel chair with a ventilator inside the house:

> Not long after we got home we figured ways of being able to manoeuvre the electric wheelchair around the house without having to move the big chair with us. I think we had a pram and we set it up underneath the pram and I think we pushed this pram around. It was one of those ones with the big wheels.

The inclusion of medical equipment and supplies in a home requires creativity and innovation particularly when trying to reduce the 'unfit' appearance of medical machines to the home (Figure 5.2). For example, there can be a need for a hospital bed to be located in a family's living room as explained by the following parent who stated that

> Because it looks a bit like a hospital, with the hospital bed and all the machines and stuff, a guy did all his bed as a big fire engine. That's why there's a big red thing at the end of his bed ... so it didn't look like a hospital bed.

Within this seemingly restrained environment promoting the child's independence as much as possible is equally important regardless of the involvement of medical technology in care. For example, being innovative enables a

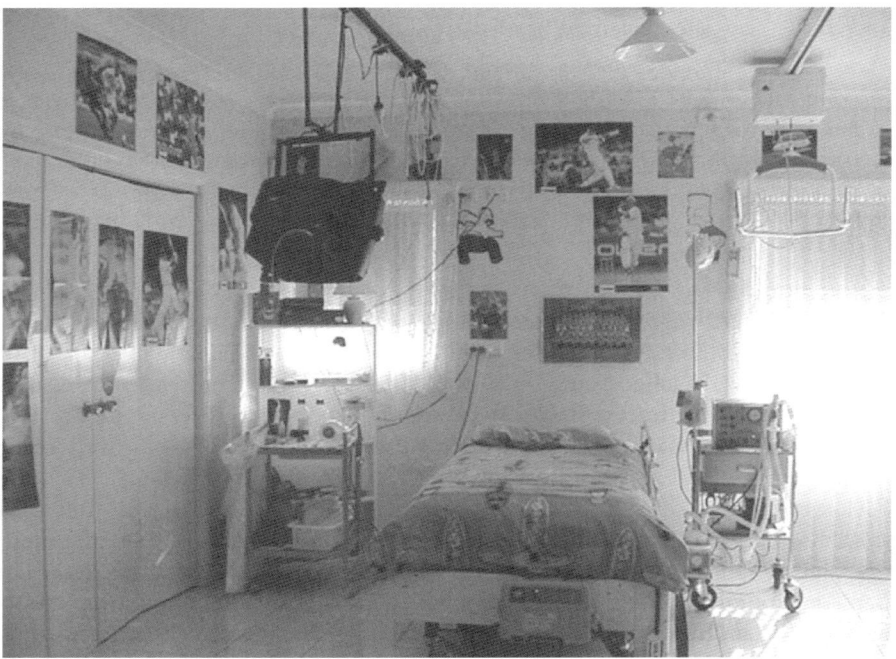

**Figure 5.2** A child's bedroom environment can often look more like an intensive care unit than a typical bedroom in the home. Note the complete absence of children's toys and furniture.

ventilator-dependent and wheel-chair-bounded child to enjoy the independence of eating an icy pole:

> When we were giving him an icy pole and he wanted to hold it himself, and I had to, with his chair, [so we] work[ed] out a way for him to do it himself. So I taped the icy pole to his chin piece so, that way he could do it himself.

### Our life is hectic!

While quality care for the technology-dependent child is of importance, care for parents and a sibling also requires extra sensitivity, because an impact of medical technology on the comfort and privacy of a home is inevitable. For instance, the alarms of a ventilator or monitor can become a source of constant stress as explained by the following father who stated that

> It was very, very hard because of the alarms ... and all the different machinery going off. It was sort of you'd get to bed and then one alarm would go off and then you'd roll over and there'd be another alarm that would go off. So, you're sort of constantly up and down, up and down.

Moreover, parents are confronted by the perpetual and often monotonous pattern of care. For example, a mother of a child who is dependent on 24 hours ventilation support was frustrated by the same tasks that she has to do every day and this is how she explained her frustration:

> Just the monotonous care day in and day out ... . I have to administer his aspirin every day ... has to have the gastrostomy tube cleaned every day and rotated to help him with his bowels ... give him a massage to help the bowels to move before his bath ... and also the oral feeding that has to be done every day ... trying to get him to stand ... to do exercises to strengthen the backs of his legs ... and interact with him to help him with his development. That's the tiring thing, the things I have to do every day.

In addition to the repetitive nature of care the level of technical skills required to perform care for a technology-dependent child is higher than those for general care. For example, one mother described the challenges of caring for a person with a tracheostomy by stating that 'the most frightening thing was the care around the tracheostomy. It's certainly a specialised field and just getting over the fear of changing them, caring for them, and the suctioning were really stressful, and it had to be done a lot.'

The nature of care of a technology-dependent child is not only medically specialised, but also more likely to result in medical emergencies that are potentially lethal to the life of the child. For example, one mother of a two-year-old baby depending on 24 hour invasive ventilation assistance reiterated the importance of collaboration with her carer in the management of an emergency called tracheostomy de-cannulation:

> We were doing a normal routine trachy change, Ann (the carer) was here, it was a Thursday, five days before Christmas ... Jane (the older sibling) was home from school on holidays by that time. We were calm. All was fine. We were getting ready, all set up to do the change. We got all the new one out, got everything organised.

Anyway, we had him elevated and on the count of three Ann takes it out and I put it in. Well, Ann took it out all right but I couldn't get it back in and I was trying so many times. So we throw that out and Ann grabbed a smaller tube that was always over the cot ... we grabbed the 3.0 and it wouldn't go in ... it was blood, there was trauma. Got a soft wick, it was the closest thing I could grab. 'Ring up quickly Jane!' Of course we were hysterical ... Ann was on the other side of the cot and she was bagging him with the bell bag and she had to keep an eye on him that he didn't go into unconsciousness in case she had to do CPR (Cardio-Pulmonary Resuscitation). We started oxygen through the Guedel bag because he was going quite blue in all the hysteria.

The work is extensive and constant when providing the medical care. One mother explained that 'he's on a monitor twenty four hours a day ... If he sleeps well, I probably get up every two hours to suction him, to feed him and turn him, and just to make sure that he's okay'.

Whilst medical care is labour intensive, care of medical equipment is also burdening and confining. For example, one mother revealed her experience of medical machinery that 'to go up the street I'd have to load the ventilator, suction units, emergency kits, and it'd be like an hour procedure just to get him up the street'.

Medical equipment is not only confining with respect to mobilising around but also limiting to daily functioning. For example, another mother described her strategy for taking a shower at night:

For many years and even now, I keep my showers to less than five minutes if I'm here on my own in case ... because you can't hear the alarm when you are in the shower. So, if you make it less than five minutes and that if he's had a vomit, you can probably resuscitate him after five minutes with some success.

### When you live at home with a ventilator-dependent child: You don't fit anywhere!

Families who care for technology-dependent children at home can experience stress not only from the demands of medical care and equipment, but also from a lack of support and understanding in the community with respect to their needs and experiences. Lack of education and understanding of the unique experiences at home of caring for a technology-dependent child can lead to mis-understanding and discrimination, which are distressing for the families: 'I didn't like it when I went to the welfare centre, because people were looking at her and pretending that we weren't there because they were too embarrassed I felt very isolated, I hated that.'

While people's misunderstanding of a families situation can result in feelings of isolation, the need to provide care that demands a range of specialised medical and technical skills is also a direct factor leading to potential isolation of parents.

After [the child] has this tracheostomy and all this equipment, I go to the shops and I'd feel like everyone was staring and wanted to know what was wrong with him but these things have actually complicated life terribly. And, the fact that if somebody says, 'can I baby-sit your child for you?', and I say, 'well he's got a tracheostomy', and then everyone says, 'well, oop!' Well then, it's just makes ME feel that he's different. And, I don't want him to ever feel that he's different.

Medical machinery, suctioning noise, tracheostomy tubes and wires not only lead to a perception that the child is different from the 'normal' child, even one who needs special cares, but also extenuate fear of being different. In addition, the stress of coping with isolation can also be exacerbated by a lack of appropriate social and health care industry support for a technology-dependent child and their family. Technology-dependent children are identifiable for both their broad range of medical diagnoses (e.g. cerebral palsy, asthma or muscular dystrophy) and for specific technologies such as artificial ventilators, suctioning equipment, resources for tracheostomy care and oxygen monitors. Accessing appropriate support for families of in-home technology-dependent children is a challenge, as explained by one mother who revealed that in her experience: 'It's really scary for us because there is no other ventilated [children in our neighbourhood], especially quadriplegics like [our ventilator-dependent child].'

Respite assistance (carers) may or may not be available, because families rely on people with specialist knowledge. The carer can be either a professional nurse or a lay caregiver but must be specifically trained in the care of the child. Care at home requires constant vigilance and attention to detail. Rotation of care-giving is necessary, and as a result of employing outside carers there are inevitable issues related to a family's privacy in their own home. For instance, one father noted that 'having someone in the house that's not part of the family and staying here overnight while you're in the bedroom two doors away, to me, that doesn't seem like support, more an inconvenience.'

Consideration and respect of a family's need for privacy are of great importance and can be improved through effective communication. One mother revealed the way her highly valued carer communicated with her: 'She always asks me before she does anything. She doesn't assume to do something with [the child] until I'm asked first. She's always checking in with me that she's done everything properly.'

Support from carers is greatly needed by families but sensitivity to the specific needs of each child and family are essential qualities of a carer, as one father explained: 'If they're to be part of the day-to-day life, I think they should try and minimise their intrusion into the family, minimise their participation into the family, try to be as inconspicuous as possible, and try to have as least impact on the family as they can.'

## 5.3 Health care and the home

In many Western countries there is increasing policy governing health care and political moves to include the community as partners in care. They have become a crucial part of health care services. There is steady increase in the numbers of patients receiving care at home. Researchers have argued that further investigation in this area is critical, especially with respect to how care associated with medical technology at home affects each person and their family. We as nurses, whether working in a hospital or the community, need to understand the experiences and needs of families so that appropriate support can be effectively formulated and provided (Heaton, et al., 2005; Kirk & Glendinning, 2004; Parette & McMahan, 2002; Wang & Barnard, 2004).

Families of in-home technology-dependent children experience 'technology' not only in relation to working with medical equipment and ordering supplies, but also in relation to personal and social experience. Technology is more than tools or equipment. Technology is associated with changes to the way we think, the way we act and our whole day (Barnard, 2002; Barnard & Sandelowski, 2001; Locsin, 2001).

Medical technology at home creates for this group of children and their families a different type of home environment. Families of technology-dependent children at home search for new meaning(s) to make sense of the changes in their lives. Medicalisation at home means people must sacrifice degrees of personal privacy and freedom, acquire specialist skills and knowledge for care, and accept what is normally foreign technology in the home. The inclusion of medical machinery can reduce usable physical space in the home and can result in inconvenience and restructuring to the geography of a house. The presence of medical equipment and 'other' carers creates restriction to mobility, may lead to confinement to a residence and an increasing sense of social isolation. Whilst discharging technology-dependent children home might reduce (or certainly shift) health care costs for a health care system and promote growth and development of a child (Fields, et al., 1991; Fusco, 1994; Kertoy, 2004; Noyes, 2000), the experiences are not without significant human cost and involve significant impact upon the meaning of a 'home', the social meaning of 'family' and relations with the community. For example, some parents of in-home ventilator-dependent children describe their situation clearly as abnormal: 'It's not like in a normal house where you've just got your normal house chores and then you relax.'

For many of us, 'home' is a place of personal comfort and privacy; however, families who care for a ventilator-dependent child at home experience 'home' with new meanings (Wang, 2005). Based on this research and a review of published evidence, better support is essential for families who care for an individual dependent on medical technology at home and should include; prompt discharge with sufficient training for carers (Glendinning & Kirk, 2000; Noyes, 2002; Noyes, et al., 1999), flexible respite (Murphy, 2001; Oslen & Maslin-Prothero, 2001), community education (Kirk, 1999), financial assistance based on individual assessment of needs (House, 1995; Roberts, 2001) and appropriate social support (Ratliffe, et al., 2002). When planning support for families of children dependent on home ventilation, health care providers must consider the level of practical support needed to best meet the needs of each individual and family.

## 5.4 Final reflection

The move of people requiring significant medical technology to support their health from hospital to home should force community health teams to think about practice in new and different ways. While use of medical technology in hospital focuses on health care professionals in the care of critically ill patients, use of medical technology in the community requires a focus on assisting to maintain family stability and promote quality of life for each person caring for a child. Early hospital discharge has resulted in an increased number of patients and their families choosing to take on the responsibility of performing medical care at home. Health care professionals working in the community must understand the influence of medical technology on the lives of these people and organise appropriate support to meet the needs of families who care for a technology-dependent child at home.

Technology is clearly not only about the task of using medical supplies and machinery, but is linked directly to personal and social values and relationships. Although the hardware and function of medical technology can be easily seen and attracts our attention, the value and need to support human dignity should not be overlooked at the expense of what is obvious about care. Further research and evidence is needed urgently so that education, support and practice can be appropriately developed to provide increased help to care for technology-dependent children in the community.

### LEARNING ACTIVITIES

1. Identify a website directed to carers of people in the community. Evaluate the quality of information with respect to currency, readability and usefulness from the consumer's perspective.

2. Survey a person in your neighbourhood about their perception of caring for people in the community. Are there specific issues they raise about community care and how well do they understand issues related to supporting the person, their carers and the family? Report your findings and thoughts to the group.

3. Form two small groups and debate the advantages and disadvantages of caring for ventilated children at home. List the key issues raised during the debate and determine strategies to address them.

## References

Barnard, A. (2002). Philosophy of technology and nursing. *Nursing Philosophy, 3*(1), 15–26.

Barnard, A. & Sandelowski, M. (2001). Technology and human nursing care: (Ir)Reconcilable or invented difference? *Journal of Advanced Nursing, 34*(3), 367–375.

Barnard, A., McCosker, H. & Gerber, R. (1999). Phenomenography: A qualitative research approach for exploring understanding in healthcare. *Qualitative Health Research, 9*(2), 212–226.

Dahlgren, L. O. & Fallsberg, M. (1991). Phenomenography as a qualitative approach in social pharmacy research. *Journal of Social and Administrative Pharmacy, 8*(4), 150–157.

Edgü, E. & Ünlü, A. (2003). Relation of domestic space preferences with Space Syntax parameters. proceedings, *4th International Space Syntax Symposium.* 17–19 June, London.

Fields, A. L., Rosenblatt, A., Pollack, M. M. & Kaufman, J. (1991). Home care cost-effectiveness for respiratory technology-dependent children. *American Journal of Diseases of Children,* *145*(7), 729–733.

Fusco, R. (1994). Home care: An emerging solution to the healthcare crisis. *Hospital Topics,* *72*(4), 32–36.

Glendinning, C. & Kirk, S. (2000). High-tech care: high skilled parents. *Paediatric Nursing,* *12*(6), 25–27.

Heaton, J., Noyes, J., Sloper, P. & Shah, R. (2005). Families' experiences of caring for technology-dependent children: a temporal perspective. *Health and Social Care in the Community,* *13*(5), 441–450.

House, J. L. (1995). *Paediatric Home Care: The Labor Contribution of Informal System Caregivers Who Forego Earnings to Care for Ventilator-dependent Children.* Thesis. Doctor of Philosophy. University of Pennsylvania.

Kirk, S. (1999). Caring for children with specialised healthcare needs in the community: The challenges for primary care. *Health and Social Care in the Community,* *7*(5), 350–357.

Kirk, S. & Glendinning, C. (2004). Developing services to support parents caring for a technology-dependent child at home. *Child: Care, Health and Development,* *30*(3), 209–219.

Kertoy, M. K. (2004). Preparing professionals for the challenge of children who are technology dependent: understanding and meeting the social and emotional needs of families. *Journal of Speech-Language Pathology and Audiology,* *28*(3), 132–141.

Locsin, R. C. (2001). Practicing nursing: Technological competency as an expression of caring. In Locsin, R. C. (ed.), *Advancing Technology, Caring, and Nursing.* Westport, CT: Auburn House, pp. 88–95.

Marton, F. (1981). Phenomenography-describing conceptions of the world around us. *Instructional Science,* *10,* 177–200.

Marton, F. (1986). Phenomenography: A research approach to investigating different understandings of reality. *Journal of Thought,* *21*(3), 28–49.

Marton, F. (1988). Phenomenography: Exploring different conceptions of reality. In Fetterman, D. (ed.), *Qualitative Approaches to Evaluation in Education: The Silent Revolution.* New York: Praeger, pp. 176–205.

Marton, F. (2000). The structure of awareness. In Bowden, J. A. & Walsh, E. (eds) *Phenomenography.* Melbourne: RMIT Publishing, pp. 102–116

Marton, F. & Booth, S. (1997). *Learning and Awareness.* New Jersey, NJ: Lawrence Erlbaum Associates.

Miles, M. S., Holditch-Davis, D., Burchinal, P. & Nelson, D. (1999). Distress and growth outcomes in mothers of medically fragile infants. *Nursing Research,* *48*(3), 129–140.

Murphy, G. (2001). The technology-dependent child at home part 2: The need for respite. *Paediatric Nursing* *13*(8), 24–28.

Noyes, J. (2000). Ventilator-dependent' children who spend prolonged periods of time in intensive care units when they no longer have a medical need or want to be there. *Journal of Clinical Nursing,* *9*(5), 774–783.

Noyes, J. (2002). Barriers that delay children and young people who are dependent on mechanical ventilators from being discharged from hospital. *Journal of Clinical Nursing,* *11*(1), 2–11.

Noyes, J., Hartmann, H., Samuels, M. & Southall, D. (1999). The experiences and views of parents who care for ventilator-dependent children. *Journal of Clinical Nursing,* *8*(4), 440–450.

Oslen, R. & Maslin-Prothero, P. (2001). Dilemmas in the provision of own-home respite support for parents of young children with complex healthcare needs: Evidence from an evaluation. *Issues and Innovations in Nursing Practice,* *34*(5), 603–610.

Parette P. & McMahan, G. A. (2002). What should we expect of Assistive Technology? Being sensitive to family goals. *Teaching Exceptional Children, 35*(1), 56–61.

Ratliffe, C. E., Harrigan, R. C., Haley, J., Tse, A. & Olsoon, T. (2002). Stress in families with medically fragile children. *Issues in Comprehensive Pediatric Nursing, 25*(1), 167–188.

Reed, C. (1996). Introduction. In Reed, C. *Not At Home: The Suppression of Domesticity in Modern Art and Architecture* (1st edn.). New York: Thames & Hudson, pp. 7–17.

Roberts, G. (2001). Supporting children with serious healthcare needs: Analyzing the costs and benefits. *Evaluation and the Health Professions, 24*(1), 72–83.

Stephenson, C. (1999). Well-being of families with healthy and technology-assisted infants in the home: A comparative study. *Journal of Pediatric Nursing, 14*, 164–176.

Thyen, U., Kuhlthau, K. & Perrin, J. M. (1999). Employment, child care and mental health of mothers caring for children assisted by technology. *Pediatrics, 103*(6) Pt 1, 1235–1242.

Wang, K. W. K. (2005). Understanding the experiences of primary caregivers who care for a ventilator-dependent child at home. PhD Thesis. Queensland University of Technology, Australia, Australian Digital Thesis (ADT).

Wang, K. W. K. & Barnard, A. (2004). Technology-dependent children and their families: A review. *Journal of Advanced Nursing, 45*(1), 36–46.

## RECOMMENDED READING

Votroubek, W. L. & Townsend, J. L. (1997). *Pediatric Home Care* (2nd edn.). Maryland: Aspen Publishers.

Wang, K. W. K. & Barnard, A. (2004). Technology-dependent children and their families: A review. *Journal of Advanced Nursing, 45*(1), 36–46.

# Robots and Nursing: Concepts, Relationships and Practice

Aric Campling, Tetsuya Tanioka and Rozzano Locsin

## LEARNING OBJECTIVES

When you have read this chapter, you will be able to:

- Describe the difference between robots, robotics and nursing systems

- Trace the historical development and functions of robots

- Describe robotic features that raise critical issues on the utilisation of robots in nursing and health care.

- Explain key issues and concepts significant to understanding robots and nursing systems

- State the theoretical underpinnings of robotics technology and their impact on future research, theory development and clinical nursing practice.

## KEY WORDS

- caring

- nursing

- robots

- robotics

- technological competency

## 6.1 Introduction

Robot is a word that according to the *American Heritage Dictionary of the English Language* (2000) was first used in the modern sense by the Czech writer Karel Capek. Capek wrote a play called Rossum's Universal Robots, in which mechanical beings were engineered specifically to function as labourers. The word originates from the Czech word robota, which means 'drudgery' or 'servitude' (Jerz, 2002). The concept of the robot, that is a humanoid automaton not made of flesh and blood, is as old as Greek mythology. Hephaestus, the Greek God of fire and the forge, created several beings from metal, including the bronze giant Talos who circled the island of Crete and protected its shores (Asimov, 1977). This chapter focuses on description of machines with humanlike characteristics and of human beings with technological parts; and clarification of the practice of nursing as involving technological expertise. The chapter includes a critical overview of the utilisation of robots in nursing, the resultant issues inherent in the use of robots in nursing and particular applications in clinical practice. Taken into consideration is a balanced and considered look at the outcomes of robot utilisation and patient-care systems with particular focus on available evidence relating to current practice and implications for continued change. Exemplars are included to guide, instruct and provide opportunities for the reader within the context and focus of the chapter, which is to understand the issues of technology, robotics and nursing.

## 6.2 Robots and robotics

A robot is typically understood to be a mechanical device that has motion, form and performs automated, complicated tasks by means of artificial intelligence (AI). That is, a robot is mechanical and reprogrammable technology controlled by a computer, and equipped with sensors and actuators to allow it to interact with its environment in a meaningful way. Robotics, a term coined in 1941 by Isaac Asimov (1979), refers to the coming together of various science and engineering disciplines that leads to an understanding of and appreciation for automated machinery. Robotics is a comprehensive science that includes learning about the structure and function of the human body, as well as the various social, cognitive and behavioural sciences.

The twentieth century was a period primed for the development of robot mechanisms. Breakthroughs in engineering studies enabled the development of machines that could closely imitate human movement. In part, advances in robotics have also arisen from advances in personal technology. Personal computers and the Internet, for instance, have made possible communication and collaboration on a worldwide scale (Kiuchi, 1999). Increases in computer processing power and data-storage enables engineers to design increasingly complex robotic mechanisms and programs to drive them in industries that rely on production line automation.

Benefits from engineering as a technology of 'things' have been, for example, convenience, comfort, safety, reliability and satisfaction. Robot technology developed today continues to be applied to industrial robotics, including intellectual robots (thinking machines) with operational abilities coming closer to that of humans (Nakagawa & Ito, 2005). In addition, robotic engineering is now undergoing increasing transition towards developing better human technology. The aims of this transition are adaptation to the environment and co-existence with humans. At the same time the type of robot required or demanded by society is shifting from the one that enables efficient productivity to a new type that can adapt to human life or society. Common understanding that a robot is a machine is changing slowly as the appearance and movement of some robots are now human-like.

Robots have been strongly represented in science fiction. American and European fiction involving robots typically describes grim scenarios where robots evolve beyond their creators, realise their potential superiority and attempt to eradicate or gain control over humanity (Asimov, 1979; Brooks, 2002). For example, the robots in *The Matrix* enslaved humanity and used them as energy sources; the main character in the *Terminator* is sent back in time to ensure that robots would one day take over the world. In order to pre-empt these types of events, the writer Isaac Asimov developed his three laws of robotics (1979). Even today, robot engineers and programmers take these laws seriously, even though they were created as a work of fiction. The Three Laws of Robotics are

1. A robot may not injure a human being, or, through inaction, allow a human being to come to harm.

2. A robot must obey orders given it by human beings, except where such orders would conflict with the First Law.

3. A robot must protect its own existence as long as such protection does not conflict with the First or Second Laws. (Asimov 1979)

Asimov asserts that these laws should be built into their programming by humans. In fact, these laws, their interpretation and subtle logical inconsistencies are often the cause of central conflicts depicted in fiction (Brooks, 2002). In 1979 Asimov understood that a robot did not have the processing power to recognise what a human was, or to have enough of a self-concept to obey even the strictest or simplest interpretation of the three laws of robotics. Brooks confirms this to still be the case but some modern robots such as Kismet (Brazeal, 2002) have the capacity to recognise a human face. Notwithstanding, robot engineers and programmers have yet to design a perceptual and cognitive system capable of handling all of the subtleties and nuances implied by the Three Laws of Robotics. The challenge does not prevent them from trying to come closer to that goal.

In contrast to an antagonistic view of robots which prevails in American and European fiction, Japanese society accepts robots as friends or allies in society and even as family members. Perspectives and theories of robotics in Japan can be traced back to an ancient art form known as wind-up doll (Karakuri Ningyo). The art of Karakuri involved hidden mechanisms in dolls or puppets that allowed these devices to perform specific, autonomous tasks. An example would be a doll designed to serve tea to a guest when a cup is placed in its hands. Another is an archer puppet which shoots arrows at a target. The puppet is designed intentionally to miss the target one out of ten times (Boyle, 2003b) in order to lend to the robot a sense of human fallibility.

Central to Karakuri is a design that conceals technology and emphasises a less life-like appearance. Western culture prefers the formation of puppets that are often designed with movable facial features in order to show expressions to observers. This design tradition carries over into modern robotics such as Kismet (Boyle, 2003a; Brazeal, 2002). In Karakuri design, faces are solid carvings and are designed to utilise shadow and lighting to convey changing expressions (Boyle, 2003a). The sense that all things have a spirit – even inanimate objects – is visible in the Japanese approach to robotics (Boyle, 2003a). Movement, was attributed to such spirits, and today, the Karakuri tradition can be seen in robots such as the Honda ASIMO or Sony QRIO robots. Both are very close to human in movement and form but have solid almost featureless faces.

## 6.3  Theories regarding robotics

For this chapter there are two robot types of interest: Remote-presence robots and autonomous robots. Remote-presence robots function within, and may even interact with the environment, but the robot's operator is not in the same room, building or even country (Brooks, 2002). Remote-presence robots are typically designed with complex AI routines that receive simple commands and translate them into discrete tasks. This way, the user of the robot does not need to worry about the intricacies of how their robot will perform a task; they give the robot an instruction, such as 'move across the room', and its AI programming will figure out the best way to achieve the desired outcome. Users are still required to direct the robot from a remote console in real-time, for instance, via a web-page with controls and a camera image (Brooks, 2002).

Autonomous robots are similar, in that the robot's programmer does not need to be in the same area as the robot operates. The robot is programmed (or pre-programmed) to perform a task or set of tasks and then is set on its way. The difference to a remote-presence robot is that the autonomous robot will not need to take further instruction until the larger task, such as vacuuming a room or mowing a lawn, is complete (Brooks, 2002). Some take no additional instruction at all. Autonomous robots frequently have built in self-maintenance routines like returning to a power outlet to recharge or avoiding the edge of a staircase. Remote-presence robots do have certain autonomous aspects about them, especially since the programming involved is very similar. In fact, many robots are both autonomous and remote-presence at once or can switch between the two as needed.

In order for any robot to function in the physical world, it must meet two requirements: It must be socially situated and it must be embodied (Brazeal, 2002). A situated robot is embedded in the world; that is, it deals with the world through sensors, which directly influence the behaviour of the robot (Brazeal, 2002; Brooks, 2002). Sensors obtain data pertinent to the robot's task, such as audio, video or tactile input. The input is processed by the AI programming to determine how it should react to the stimuli based on its overall function, the task it was commanded to perform and other factors.

In order to meaningfully respond to the stimulus, the robot needs a body with which to interact with its environment. An embodied robot has a physical body and experiences its environment through interactions with the body (Brazeal, 2002; Brooks, 2002). An example is the intensive-care cardiac monitor. It is situated, but not wholly embodied. The monitor has sensors allowing it to detect various vital signs required for a clinician to provide care, but the machine does not interact physically with its environment of its own accord, based on processing of the input data.

Some robots have been designed to function in a social manner, learning from and interacting with the social world. This design trend towards sociable robots is the next extension to situation and embodiment. The sociable robot acts and reacts in socially appropriate ways – the robot must learn what is socially acceptable and appropriate behaviour from its environment and be able to express its internal 'emotional' state (Brazeal, 2002). However, how will society accept robots? As robots become more adept – especially learning robots that will grow emotionally and intellectually in ways similar to children – where will the line be drawn between machine and person? (Brazeal, 2002). Will the day come when robots are fully socially aware?

## 6.4 Anthropomorphic machines

Anthropomorphism is the attribution of human characteristics to nonhumans or machines. The thought that future human beings will relate emotionally with machines is regarded often as fiction. However human beings are forming emotional relationships with partly-mechanical people. Many humans have technological parts such as pacemakers, artificial limbs, insulin pumps, metal hip joints or even mechanical hearts. Can people be considered partly machines since they are technologically dependent? What is the demarcation or boundary between human and machine? When is partly human and partly machine not a machine? If being partly human makes a person partly a machine, then a machine that perhaps has emotions, human appearance or some other anthropomorphic attributes, could be partly human! What is the distinction between human and machine?

The ability to communicate verbally is important to humans and is a prized characteristic. Car alarms blurt out sirens that seem to say 'Stand back, you are too close', and elevators sometimes announce the different levels of a building by way of pre-recorded messages. These are cues for humans that could be useful to robots who respond also to verbal stimuli. For example, the ability to respond to commands and to anticipate appropriate human behaviours are essential qualities for mechanical objects in nursing.

The sociable robot acts and reacts in socially appropriate ways. Some are machines that do tasks in factories and hospitals. Some are life-like toys. Some are digital images on the screen. In the future, autonomous mobile robots are likely to assist people in many environments. Robots may help the elderly and their caregivers with work around the home, act as guards and perform tasks that are repetitive, boring or dangerous in nursing homes, hospitals, military environments, disaster sites and schools (Carnegie Mellon University, 2004). A robot must therefore learn acceptable and appropriate social behaviour from its environment and must be able to express its internal 'emotional' state. These are challenges for the future design of robots.

## 6.5 Robotics and nursing: Knowledge for nursing in the twenty-first century and beyond

Nurses typically learn anatomy, biochemistry, physiology and other social sciences, but not the study of robotics as they pertain to health care practice. Devices built with robotic technology are widespread in community nursing and hospital environments. For instance, in the intensive-care unit, an electrocardiogram (ECG) monitor is designed to monitor the heart rate, rhythm and other vital signs of patients with circulatory instability. Ventilators that help patients breathe mechanically are used during cases of respiratory compromise. Should not nurses who use robotic technology understand the engineering behind the devices in order to ensure the safety of their human patients? It is possible to classify human functions from the engineering standpoint in the following ways: (1) Functions for survival; (2) functions for intellectual/mental activities; and (3) functions related to physical movements (Kiuchi, 1999). The engineering that supports the human life-related fields such as medicine and health management spans a continuum from medical engineering to welfare engineering. These types of engineering address life-related patterns and generate life-support technologies that sustain those who are experiencing deterioration or loss of biological functions or causing obstruction to full engagement in social activities and everyday life. The technologies of robotics and medical engineering are applied in fields such as health management, n overcoming illnesses and dysfunction, as support for comfortable living and for enabling participation in social activities (Dohi, 1999) (Figure 6.1).

In order to use robots and engineering machines with humans and human systems, approaches from the study of motion mechanisms, control, measurement and information processing are applied to hardware designs. Since robot technology will interact with, or apply to humans, an approach from the field of biomedical engineering is also warranted. Biomimetics is one such field, and is the use of living systems as inspiration for machines (Menzel & D'Aluisio, 2000). The field is seeking to inspire the design of robots with flexible mechanisms and the development of micro-robotics.

Software approaches for moving robots have usually been the domain of AI; in fact, some of the largest AI labs have produced the most prominent robots in the field. The study of biological, psychological and sociological aspects are all essential to the creation of robots. Moreover, appropriate approaches are crucial in addressing concerns related to psychology, emotion and sensitivity engineering of robots.

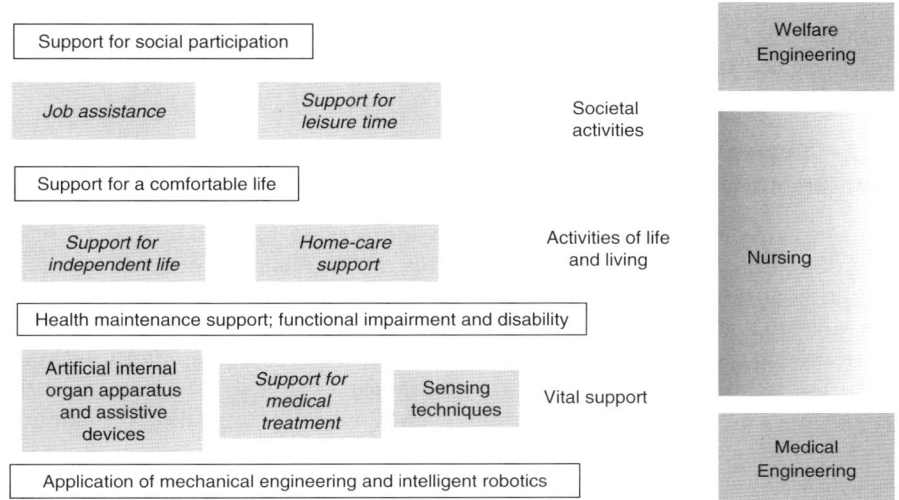

**Figure 6.1** Life support technology and nursing care (Dohi T, 1999). Tanioka adapted the Dohi figure for use in nursing.

## 6.6 Robotics in nursing

We must be fully aware of the situations in which social phenomena and changes in ethical approaches are warranted because of the introduction of robots for supporting humans in health care situations of everyday life. It is necessary to integrate knowledge of robot technologies in order to improve the quality of life of patients and users alike. In doing so, it is essential to consider what is sharable knowledge (including skills) and how interdisciplinary communication between users such as doctors, nurses, engineers, entrepreneurs and health care managers should be enhanced. Nurses must be involved in the process of considering the applications of robotics in care. Quite simply, the acquisition of knowledge related to robotics is helpful to nurses when using such devices to care for patients. For instance, when using a ventilator, a nurse should be able to consider the physiological mechanisms that inform nursing technologies like understanding the relationship of the setup of pressure-assisted respirations, danger avoidance functions and human intra-alveolar pressure.

Moreover, nurses are well suited to consider the desirable functions of a machine from the perspective of the patient. Nurses are able to cooperate with engineers in developing devices necessary for enhancing nursing care and to propose improvements of biomedical and robotic devices for the purpose of enhancing care. Unless an engineer has some knowledge about physiology, anatomy, sociology and psychology, it is impossible to best develop a device for human care. Similarly, if nurses cannot explain the functions required of a machine to assist with patient care, it is difficult for an engineer to develop or improve upon such a device. A common knowledge and language at a level that enables interdisciplinary communication between specialists is an essential development of technological competency in nursing.

## 6.7 Types and uses of robots in health care institutions

Autonomous robots are used widely in industry in the production of many technological goods. Assembly-line robots do the majority of work in manufacturing automobiles – for example, robots can be used in dangerous areas or for work that requires repetition or precision. Advanced application of robotics in health care is still a relatively young field but it has several applications in the industry. In some hospitals it is common to see a robot delivering medications to nursing units (wards) or wandering in a hospital collecting laboratory samples and delivering them.

### Example:

A 362-bed community hospital in Boynton Beach, Florida, utilises courier robots that deliver medication from the pharmacy to the nursing units. 'ReX' sits outside the pharmacy and waits for an instruction to 'go'. The pharmacist loads medications into the robot's compartment, and pushes a few buttons to set the robot rolling.

Health care facilities such as telehealth also assist doctors and surgeons to assess patients and perform intricate surgery from thousands of miles away through the assistance of robotics. The role of robots in health care can be divided into three discrete categories:

- Passive role: The role of the passive-role robot is limited in scope with largely low risk involvement.

- Restricted role: The restricted role robot is responsible for more invasive tasks with higher risk but is still restricted from essential portions of the procedure.

- Active role: The active-role robot is intimately involved in the procedure and carries high responsibility and risk. (Camarillo, Krummel & Salisbury, 2004)

### Clinical examination and diagnosis

Clinical examination and diagnosis encompasses functions such as magnetic resonance imaging (MRI) scan, computed tomography (CT) and more. Generally, these are passive-role robots. Complex AI systems combined with 3-dimensional CT imaging that apply intelligent diagnostic algorithms to images of breast tissue with the intent of improving accuracy of the diagnosis of cancer even at early stages are under investigation (Lo, 2005). CT in general is an imaging modality that uses manipulation of gathered data to clarify scanner images by means of actuators, sensors and processors. Therefore, some surgical applications that use CT are considered robot-assisted systems, but they require detailed attention to the technology itself to realise this as an exemplary application of robotics to surgery (Camarillo, Krummel & Salisbury, 2004).

## Medical treatment

Medical treatment robots are increasingly taking an active role in care. Microsurgery techniques, endoscopic and laparoscopic-assisted surgery, and radiosurgery are examples of medical treatment where robots are making inroads. For example, robotics offers a unique approach to radiosurgery, a process that uses pinpoint targeting of radiation to operate non-invasively on lesions (particularly in the brain) (Adler, et al., 1997; University of Florida, 2005). Rather than using rigid immobilisation of the patient, this process relies on AI interpretation and correlation of fluoroscopy and CT images to localise its target. First, the robot stops at a programmed point and fluoroscopy is conducted. The pictures obtained from the robot's camera and from the CT scans are compared, from which the treatment site is pinpointed. The patient's location and position is transmitted to the robot. Instead of moving the patient, the robot moves the radio-surgical device carefully towards the treatment site and then applies the radiation (Shiomi, et al., 2000).

## Rehabilitation

In rehabilitation, robots assist for example with muscle training, range of motion exercise and gait training. They assume passive or restricted roles in care. Robotic technology is increasingly used in prosthetic devices as well, which are designed to return more natural function to an amputee. The field of rehabilitation robotics encompasses artificial limbs and robotic solutions that address social, technological and emotional issues (Dario, Carrozza & Guglielmelli, 2003). Another area of rehabilitation robotics is development of assistive devices for the elderly. Numerous devices have been designed to assist the blind and frail when walking. Although traditional walking frames are effective for some people with impaired mobility, patients who have symptoms such as frozen gait or festinating gait may fall even when using the technology (Kai, et al., 2004; Tanioka, et al., 2004). Frozen gait, a symptom of Parkinsonism, and similar symptoms can be sensed mechanically by a robotic walking aid. Using a mathematical musculoskeletal model, it can predict a patient's fall (Kai, et al., 2002), and can then safely support the patient, where a traditional walking frame may have failed.

Rehabilitation robotics provides functional replacement, functional recovery and functional assistance. The robot acts as an intelligent mediator of care between the caregiver and the patient or even in place of the caregiver (Dario, Carrozza & Gugliemelli, 2003). For example, robots have been designed to offer upper-extremity mobility assistance and rehabilitation to patients affected by musculoskeletal or neurological injury or deficit. Other robots provide lower limb rehabilitation easily and safely by independently controlling the patient's hip, knee and foot joints simultaneously for exercise, therapy or support (Tanabe, et al., 2003).

The prosthesis is a very challenging aspect of rehabilitation robotics. Robotic hands are designed to restore more natural function and appearance to hand amputees (Carrozza, et al., 2004). Such prosthetics incorporate AI processes to take over reflexive controls like the ability to sense and adapt to items slipping from a person's grasp (Carrozza, et al., 2004; Dalloway, Jackson & Timmers, 1995). Intelligent orthotics or prostheses, which function almost like a human limb, have been developed (Carrozza, et al., 2004; DeLespinois & Locasio, 2005; Suga, et al., 1998). Consider the robot that compensates as an artificial leg for an above-the-knee amputee. A symbiosis exists between robot and human. The C-Leg orthosis (Figure 6.2) has a joint unit that controls knee movements using a microcomputer. The robotic prosthetic is controlled by the computer processes to understand and properly compensate automatically for the swing-phase of a person's stride. The robot also adjusts for the ground conditions, speed of walk (or run) and many other conditions. However, the person equipped with such a robot cannot feel instant emotional gratification since the metal and the microcomputer are not always covered with genuine-looking artificial skin.

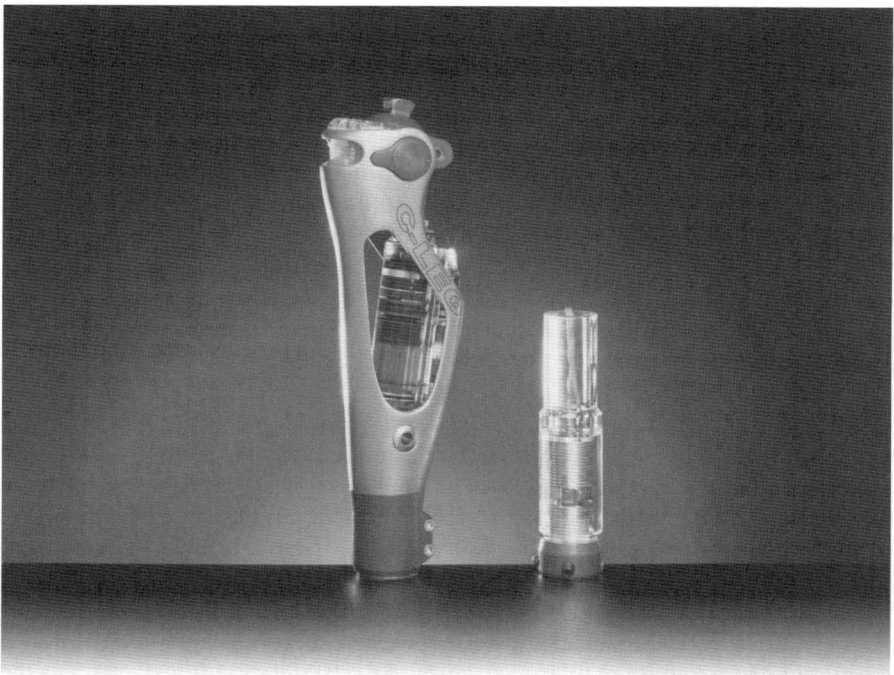

**Figure 6.2**  C-Leg Microprocessor Knee lower limb prosthesis (Copyright Otto Bock HealthCare).

## Care Assistance

Care-assist robots such as the CareBot 3.0 (Gecko Systems, 2005) (Figure 6.3) are chiefly passive-role technology and are often designed to assist patients and ensure their safety and comfort. Brooks (2002) also described a remote-presence robot used to 'check in on' elderly family members to assure their safety. CareBot 3.0 is an autonomous, embodied and situated robot with voice-recognition protocols and a complex AI that allows it to sense and avoid obstacles without veering from its task. It assists the elderly with medication or appointment reminders. CareBot 3.0 also provides a remote-presence interface allowing family members and clinicians to check on and communicate with family members through the robot. Currently in development are add-on modules that will allow CareBot 3.0 to read and act upon vital signs and other monitored patient data in a timely manner, such as by calling emergency numbers or family members (Day, 2000).

Alternative robots are being designed to assist and protect caregivers as well. One such device is a power-assisting robotic 'suit'. The suit detects the motion and load of a nurse's arms, and its mechanical joints act to augment her strength. When a woman weighing 64 kg (130 lbs) wears this suit, she can easily lift a man weighing 70 kg (154 lbs) in her arms straight up from a bed (Yamamoto, et al., 2002, 2003).

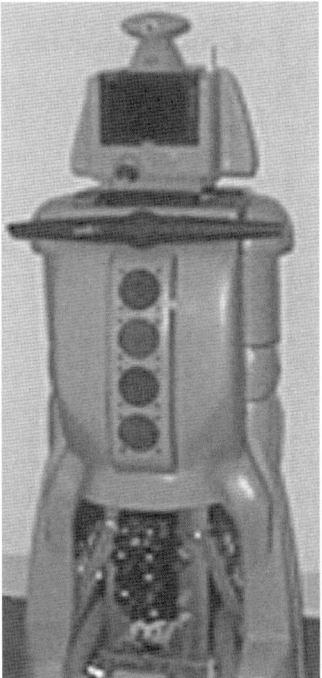

**Figure 6.3**   CareBot 3.0 (GeckoSystems. Inc).

## 6.8 Robots and health-care practitioner education

Medical and nursing education encompasses curriculum management, electronic learning and education assistance. Today, electronic learning systems monitor mandatory education requirements and can be used to learn about other topics of interest. The next generation model of interactive education support systems will utilise speech processing technology and image processing methods to determine the condition of the learner (tired, sleepy, feeling sick or well, etc.) (Lin, et al., 2006). Advice such as 'take a break, you're tired' might then be sent back to the learner in response to their perceived condition. In addition to assisting and directing the learning of individuals, robots are modelling as patients in medical and nursing schools. For instance, a simulation robot was used by one of the authors as a student at Georgetown University. Georgetown's patient simulator, SAM, could be auscultated and suctioned. It had palpable pulses and pupils that changed size based on the reactions selected by the professor. The future of educational robotics will see robots that function more autonomously. For example, an instructor will select a condition such as anaphylactic shock, and the robot will present the signs and symptoms of the condition appropriately; the student will then enter his or her treatment plan and the AI in the programming for the robot will cause the 'patient' (robot) to react in accordance with the plan.

## 6.9 Robotisation is just humanisation

Robots and the AIs that drive them are becoming increasingly complex and human-like. Robots developed in Japan have intricate joints, motors and programming that allows them to walk and move using human-like mannerisms (Brazeal, 2002; Brooks, 2002; DeLespinois & Locasio, 2005). Robots such as Kismet can successfully engage humans in social interactions. Human engineers and programmers have built robots in this familiar form for aesthetic reasons, primarily aimed towards enhancing the social acceptance of robots.

Japanese roboticist Masahiro Mori, whose study of engineering is heavily influenced by the teachings of Buddhism, posits the theory of the Uncanny Valley. This theory explains how humans react to robots and other non-human beings. The Uncanny Valley theory states that social acceptance of a robot by humans increases as the robot becomes more human-like in quality. Emotional response is increasingly positive as the robot gains more human-like qualities like movement and appearance. However, at a point where an automaton is almost nearly human-like, acceptance of the robot suddenly drops off (MacDorman, 2005), and the emotional response is one of repulsion. This is the point at which a robot is nearly human. Plotted on a graph with reaction and acceptance on the X axis and human-like quality on the Y axis, this dip in the acceptance curve is the 'Uncanny Valley' – a point at which observers find viewing or interacting with the robot disquieting or disturbing (MacDorman, 2005). As the appearance, motion and behaviour of the robot continue to be more indistinguishable than those of a human, emotional response once again rises and approaches human-to-human empathy levels.

The name Uncanny Valley harkens to the notion that a robot which is almost human seems overly strange to a human being and thus fails to evoke the requisite empathetic response required for productive human–robot interaction. Mori separately tested responses to word variations in the movement and appearance of the robot from completely machine to almost human. For both variables, the chart displayed (Figure 6.4) is a similar curve and shows the reaction.

The phenomenon can be explained by the concept that if an entity is adequately non-human-like, then the human-like characteristics will tend to stand out and be noticed easily, generating empathy. On the other hand, if the entity is almost human in appearance and behaviour, then the non-human characteristics will be the ones that stand out, leading to a feeling of strangeness and disquiet in the human viewer (Mori, 2003).

Even if the movement of a robotic arm closely resembles the motion of a human arm, a person tends not to hold the sense of belonging to industrial robots that do not resemble humans in appearance. The appearances of toy robots and the latest bipedal, humanoid robots are similar to humans and the sense of belonging increases according to the degree of similarity. However, humans feel a sense of eeriness when viewing or interacting with some robots, such as animatronic robots that are modelled on the human form using artificial skin that looks exactly like real skin (Mori, 2003).

The Sony QRIO robot (Sony Corporation, 2005) resembles a humanoid form and has sophisticated human-like movement, but is clearly mechanical or robotic in appearance (Brooks, 2002; Sony, 2005). QRIO is a 3-foot tall humanoid robot with the ability to move in a nearly human way; it recognises

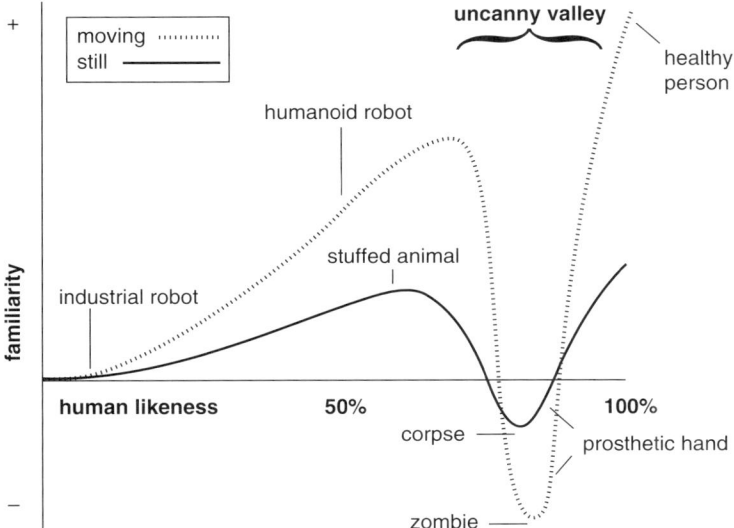

**Figure 6.4** The Uncanny Valley: Masahiro Mori graphed the relationship between human likeness and familiarity and acceptance. As human likeness increases, so does familiarity, until a point is reached where the changing differences in appearance are enough to cause an unsettling effect (Mori, as cited in MacDorman, 2005).

faces and can engage in a conversation with you. However, because its appearance is not distinctly like a human it is less likely to cause an unsettling feeling for people when watching or interacting with the robot.

A robot that can share memories from childhood and become the partner of a human being's life will someday be within the reach of humanoid robot development. Certainly, this concept is very prevalent in the entertainment industry, especially in Japan, where robots are already viewed as friends of society. At such a level, the robot is no longer a disposable thing or a tool. A robot may one day raise a child or lament a person's death. Robots may some day honestly sympathise with people. Even today, robots and humans form close symbiotic relationships. Humans are already entering a post-human era.

## Humanoid robotics

It is common for people to have replacement joints in their knees and hips. Screws, plates and rods supplant the skeletal system. Implanted lenses restore sight to eyes once clouded by cataracts. Pacemakers provide the electrical impulses for hearts that can no longer do so on their own. Implantable artificial cochleas bring humans even closer to post-humanity by providing a direct connection between the electronics of the device with the human central nervous system (Brooks, 2002). Work is also underway in many places on retinal implants, capable of restoring sight to people blinded by diseases such as macular degeneration (Brooks, 2002).

Mori (1981, 1985) explains that a humanoid robot, or a robot meant to interact with humans, cannot be designed without first understanding human beings. This understanding should not be limited to anatomy or physiology. An effort to build a robot and make it function in human-like ways is an expression of our desire to understand the human condition. Mori calls this attempt to appreciate human instinct 'philosophical anthropology' (1985, p. 4). Work with robots will only be successful if the suitability of a work environment or a task for automation is clarified. For this reason, it is important to automate a workplace based on ideas and input from workers. For instance, ReX the robot who delivers medications from the pharmacy was not introduced to the aforementioned hospital in order to save the hospital money through not paying wages. ReX was introduced to fill a task suitable for automation: that is, deliver medications so humans can do more important work. Adding robots to the workplace should support the hard work of employees and the automation handed to the robots. Therefore, it is important for employees to do their best and to plan the most appropriate work for their robots so they can do their best as well (Mori, 1985).

## Symbiosis: Robotics and the teachings of Buddhism

Phantom limb pain is a noxious and painful sensation. For a period of time a person can still feel as if a limb is attached to their body after it has been amputated. Phantom pain is a pain felt not at the edge of the amputation but at locations often more distal, such as the fingertips of an above-the-elbow amputee. It is important to understand these human sensations and feelings in perfecting the creation of robots. Particularly, it is necessary to program into a robot's 'brain' the design or model of its own body so it can identify the location and placement of all such parts (Mori, 1987). In robotics, the most difficult thing to design and implement is the physical contact between human and robot. While a human being can follow a machine as its partner, a machine will have difficulty following a human being, unless high-definition controls suitable for the human-machine interface are built into the robot. When this control cannot be executed, the robot may wound its human user, or the person may break the robot. For instance, the C-leg (Figure 6.2) could topple its user if the human-robot interface is not well-implemented. Mori (1998) highlights this mutual dependence when he quotes two short lines from the teachings of Dogen Zenji, the founder of Soto Zen Buddhism which stresses that as humans we should seek to consider all things in the world as part of our body: 'To learn about one self is to forget one self. To forget one self is to perceive one self as all things.'

## 6.10  Artificial emotions and evocative objects

How will nursing be practiced in the future now that human beings are increasingly part machine? As claimed by Sherry Turkle:

> What has become increasingly clear … is that, counter intuitively, [human beings] become attached to sophisticated machines not for their smarts but their emotional reach. They seduce [human beings] by asking for human nurturance, not intelligence. [Humans] are suckers not for realism but for relationships. (Allis, 2004, para. 4)

Nursing theory stresses human beings should be considered as whole and complete and that nursing is a process enacted between the nurse and the one nursed. Theory stresses appreciation of health as quality of life. Appreciation of these concepts clearly illustrates how nursing seeks to be recognised, how it is practised and why nursing is integral to quality health care. The focus of nursing is the person. Through the lens of Nursing as Caring, all persons are understood as caring by virtue of their humanness (Boykin & Schoenhofer, 2001). Technological advances, especially in modern medical and nursing practice, continue to challenge our definitions of person. As human beings move closer towards being 'post human', nursing theory must be flexible enough to accommodate new understandings of persons. That is, as modern and future advances in technology push towards our technological evolution, we will see cybernetic organisms (cyborgs) and other techno-sapiens – partly human beings and partly human machines – as recipients of, or partners in, nursing. What will this nursing be? How will nursing be experienced by the nurse and the one nursed?

## 6.11  Final reflection: Working and responding best to robotics

The understanding that anthropomorphic machines (Locsin, Tanioka & Kawanishi, 2005) and technological competence are linked to the practice of nursing is timely and significant. Adapting engineering technology to nursing and health care can be difficult. In higher-learning institutions it will be necessary to educate future generations of engineers and health care workers such as nurses about diagnoses, medical treatment, health care, rehabilitation and patient welfare support using robotics. Moreover, in the case of clinical nursing, fostering a positive attitude towards new technology, knowledge and research will be indispensable. Nurses have to learn the collaborative skills necessary to communicate with experts from a wide variety of backgrounds. In addition, nurses have to cultivate the capability to apply acquired knowledge into nursing practice correctly and effectively so that patient safety, comfort and well-being is enhanced. Not only that, the well-being and safety of clinicians using the technology must be ensured. Most importantly, the nurse who practices nursing as caring and understands the technological competence required to do so, will have sensitivity necessary to understand the experience of those treated through the use of robotics.

## LEARNING ACTIVITIES

1. As a group, discuss your understanding of the concept of a robot.

2. Debate the importance of anthropomorphism and sociability as they apply to the creation of robots designed to function in the various nursing areas discussed in the text. For example, is it important that a robot can look, speak, think and/or act like a human being? Would an older person feel better about being cared for by a robot with human features? Is form or function more important and to what degree?

3. In small groups identify nursing and other tasks in health care environments that could be delegated to robots. In the larger group, share your assessment of appropriate tasks for robots and the rationale for your decisions.

4. What is our understanding of person? Discuss the following quotation which asks, 'if we as nurses cannot appreciate the post-human as person, how can we adequately care for them'?

## References

Adler, J. R. Jr, Chang, S. D., Murphy, M. J., Doty, J., Geis, P., & Hancock, S. L. (1997). The Cyberknife: A frameless robotic system for radiosurgery. *Stereotactic and Functional Neurosurgery, 69*(1–4 Pt 2), 124–128.

Allis, S. (2004). Artificial emotion. *The Boston Globe*. [Retrieved 30 August 2005] http://www.boston.com/news/local/massachusetts/articles/2004/02/29/artificial_emotion/

*American Heritage Dictionary of the English Language* (2000). (4th edn.). [Retrieved 10 July 2005] http://dictionary.reference.com/search?q=robot

Asimov, I. (1977). *The Friends We Make*. Reprinted in Asimov, I. (1991). Robot Visions. New York: ROC.

Asimov, I. (1979). *The Laws of Robotics*. Reprinted in Asimov, I. (1991). Robot Visions. New York: ROC.

Boyle, K. (2003a). Robot Perspectives. [Retrieved 24 July 2005] http://www.karakuri.info/perspectives/

Boyle, K. (2003b). *Zashiki Karakuri*. [Retrieved 24 July 2005] http://www.karakuri.info/zashiki/

Boykin, A., and Schoenhofer, S. (2001). *Nursing as caring: A Model for Transforming Practice*. Sudbury, CT: Jones and Bartlett.

Brazeal, C. (2002). *Designing Sociable Robots*. Cambridge, MA: The MIT Press.

Brooks, R. A. (2002). *Flesh and Machines: How Robots Will Change Us*. New York: Pantheon Books.

Camarillo, D. B., Krummel, T. M. & Salisbury, J. K. (2004). Robotic technology in surgery: Past, present, and future. *The American Journal of Surgery, 188* (October Suppl.), 2S–15S.

Carnegie Mellon University. (2004). *Project on People and Robots*. [Retrieved 23 April 2005] http://www.peopleandrobots.org

Carrozza, M. C., Suppo, C., Sebastiani, F., Massa, B., Vecchi, F., Lazzarini, L., et al. (2004). The SPRING hand: Development of a self-adaptive prosthesis for restoring natural grasping. *Autonomous Robots, 16*(2), 125–141.

Dalloway, J. L., Jackson, R. D. & Timmers, P. H. A. (1995). Rehabilitation robotics in Europe. *IEEE Transactions on Rehabilitation Engineering, 3*, 35–45. [Retrieved 27 July 2005] http://homepage.ntlworld.com/dallaway/papers/tre95.html

Dario, P., Carrozza, M. C. & Gugliemelli, E. (2003). Guest editorial: special issue on rehabilitation robotics. *Autonomous Robots, 15*(1), 5–6.

Day, R. (1 September 2000). *Robots. Popular Mechanics*. [Retrieved 10 July 2005] http://www.popularmechanics.com/science/robotics/1282366.html

DeLespinois, P. & Locasio, F. (Executive Producers). (2005). (May 22). *The Science of Star Wars: Man and Machine*. [Television Broadcast]. Silver Spring, MD: Discovery Communications, Inc.

Dohi, T. (1999). Role of Precision Engineering in Medicine and Technical Aids, Precision Engineering, (Japanese language), *65*(4), 489–492.

GeckoSystems. (n.d.) *CareBot*™ *MSR 3.0*. [Retrieved 10 July 2005] http://www.geckosystems.com/products/carebot3.php

Jerz, D. G. (2002). R. U. R. (Rossum's Universal Robots). [Retrieved 10 July 2005] http://jerz.setonhill.edu/resources/RUR/

Kai, Y., Tanioka, T., Inoue, Y., Matuda, T., Sugawara, K., Ishida, K., et al. (2002). Prevention of a patient's falling by using a sensor controlled ambulation support machine: Analysis of leg muscle action based on the musculoskeletal model. Proceedings of *ACMD'02, The First Asian Conference on Multibody Dynamics*. 31 July–2 August, Iwaki City, Japan. 86–96.

Kai, Y., Tanioka, T., Inoue, Y., Matuda, T., Sugawara, K., Takasaka, Y., et al. (2004). A walking support/evaluation machine for patients with parkinsonism, *The Journal of Medical Investigation, 51*(1–2), 117–124.

Kiuchi, M. (1999). Development of human function and ability support engineering, some applications in manufacturing field. *Seisan Kenkyu [Industrial Research]* (Japanese language), *51*(3), 99–104.

Lin, Y., Tanioka, T., Tanihira, K., Ren, F., Tada, T., Howard, K., et al. (2006). An interactive e-learning system for practicing team care by interdisciplinary collaboration, *Kawasaki Journal of Medical Welfare, 12*(1), 37–44.

Lo, J. Y. (2005). *3D Tomosynthesis Imaging of the Breast; Computer-aided Detection/Diagnosis*. [Retrieved 11 December 2005] http://deckard.duhs.duke.edu/~jyl/bme.html

Locsin, R. C., Tanioka, T. & Kawanishi, C. (2005). Anthropomorphic machines and the practice of nursing: Knowing persons as whole in the moment. Proceedings of the *IEEE International Conference on Natural Language Processing and Knowledge Engineering (IEEE NLP-KE 2005)*, 825–829, Wuhan, China. (30 October–1 November).

MacDorman, K. F. (2005). Androids as an experimental apparatus: Why is there an Uncanny Valley and can we exploit it? Proceedings of the *CogSci-2005 Workshop*, 25–26 July, Stresa,

Italy. [Retrieved 28 August 2005] http://www.androidscience.com/proceedings2005/MacDormanCogSci2005.pdf

Menzel, P. & D'Aluisio, F. (2000). *Robo Sapiens*. Cambridge, MA: MIT Press.

Mori, M. (1981). *The Buddha in the Robot* (Japanese language). Tokyo, Japan: Kosei Publishing.

Mori, M. (1985). *Introduction to Buddhism, Quest for Human Truth From Robotics Perspective* (Japanese language), Mikasa Shobo Co., Ltd., Tokyo.

Mori, M. (1987). Robots and psychology – On the three sections, *Journal of Social Psychology* (Japanese language), 1–6.

Mori, M. (1998). Robot for happiness (Japanese language), *Journal of the Robotics Society of Japan, 16*(1), 33–36.

Mori, M. (2003). The door to creation of a robot doctor; Uncanny Valley; The cautions to human type robot design. *ROBOKON Magazine, 28*, 49–51.

Nakagawa, E. & Ito, M. (2005). *Introduction to Robotics* (Japanese language). Tokyo: Seizando Shoten.

Shiomi, H., Inoue, T., Nakamura, S., & Inoue, T. (2000). Quality assurance for an image-guided frameless radiosurgery system using radiochromic film. *Radiation Medicine, 2*(18), 107–113.

Sony Corporation (2005). *QRIO.* [Retrieved 31 July 2005] http://www.sony.net/SonyInfo/QRIO/

Suga, T., Kameyama, O., Ogawa, R., Matsuura, M. & Oka, H. (1998). Newly designed computer controlled knee-ankle-foot orthosis (intelligent orthosis). *Prosthetics and Orthotics International, 22*(3), 230–239.

Tanioka, T., Kai Y., Matsuda T., Inoue Y., Sugawara K., Takasaka Y., et al. (2004). Real-time measurement of frozen gait in patient with parkinsonism using a sensor-controlled walker. *The Journal of Medical Investigation, 51*(1–2), February, 108–116.

Tanabe, S., Sugawara, K., Tanioka, T. & Tsubahara, A. (2003). Effect of new continuous passive training device on angle and torque of knee joint. *Sogo Rehabilitation, 12*(31), 1161–1166.

University of Florida. (2005). *Understanding Stereotactic Radiosurgery.* [Retrieved 8 September 2005] http://radsurg.ufl.edu/patient/understanding.html

Yamamoto, K., Hyoudo, K., Ishii, M. & Matuo, T. (2002). Development of power assisting suit for assisting nurse labor. *The Japan Society of Mechanical Engineers International Journal, Series C1, 45*(3), 703–711.

Yamamoto, K., Hyoudo, K., Ishii, M. & Matuo, T. (2003). Development of power assisting suit for assisting nurse labor: Miniaturization of supply system to realize wearable suit. *The Japan Society of Mechanical Engineers International Journal, Series C, 46*(3), 923–930.

## RECOMMENDED READING

Brazeal, C. (2002). *Designing Sociable Robots.* Cambridge, MA: The MIT Press.

Brooks, R. (2002). *Flesh and Machines: How Robots Will Change Us.* New York: Pantheon Books.

Locsin, R. & Campling, A. (2001). Techno sapiens and posthumans: Nursing, caring, and technology. In R. Locsin, *Technological Competency as Caring in Nursing: A Model for Practice.* Indianapolis, IN: Sigma Theta Tau International Press.

Locsin, R. C. (2005). *Technological Competency as Caring in Nursing: A Model for Practice.* Sigma Theta Tau International: Indianapolis, IN.

Menzel, P. & D'Aluisio, F. (2000). *Robo Sapiens: Evolution of a New Species.* Cambridge, MA: The MIT Press.

# Telematics in Health and Nursing: The United Kingdom NHS Experience

## Paula Proctor

LEARNING OBJECTIVES

When you have read this chapter, you will be able to:

- Describe what is meant by telecare and its alternative terms
- Understand the main uses of telehealth interventions in the United Kingdom
- Consider the role nursing can play in telehealth
- Discuss the leading issues associated with telehealth and telenursing

## KEY WORDS

- education
- nursing
- policy
- technology
- telecare
- telehealth

## 7.1 'Beam me up Scotty'

As we enter the twenty-first century, our drive to harness technology to support health care is ever increasing (Mouratidis, Manson & Philp, 2003). The drive is to a large part arising from policy makers looking for non-staffing or low-staffing solutions to the maintenance of health care as demanded by the public (Thompson, 2004). Health care is a ready adopter of new technologies, sometimes with little thought as to the long-term implications for care, health professionals or the public (Barlow, Bayer & Curry, 2005).

Telematics (a global term for all things 'tele' – using a combination of visual, audio and text technologies) is one such advanced technology in health care that has received both positive and negative responses to the early adopters. The use of computers alone to support health care in the United Kingdom (UK) started in the early 1960s (Scholes, Bryant & Barber, 1982) but it was not until 1991 that telecommunications in the form of video (ISDN2 and ISDN2e) were linked allowing for one and two way video images to be used. The early adopters were anticipated to be business and commerce, through reducing time spent travelling to and from meetings, and certainly there was some interest in this use, however, other uses started to be tried, such as teledermatology. The drive to support dermatology through telematics was in part due to a poor record by general physicians in their diagnosis of dermatological conditions. With teledermatology, a video linked consultation could take place quickly and thus giving a diagnosis more effectively for treatment to commence. There are a plethora of examples of teledermatology in the early days of telemedicine, but the interest has reduced today and been overtaken by such uses as teleradiology, telenursing and teletriage. It must not be forgotten that just as we watch television in two dimensions, teledermatology used two dimensions and often for differential diagnosis three dimensions are needed along with odour, discharge and skin changes – these cannot be transmitted through technology available today.

We seem to forget that the World Wide Web (www) as we know it today only came into general use in 1994 and the increase in users is staggering, according to the National Statistics Omnibus Survey (NSOS, 2005): 'In the fourth quarter of 2004, 52 per cent of households in the UK (12.6 million) could access the Internet from home, compared with just 9 per cent (2.2 million) in the same quarter of 1998.'

The speed of public engagement with telecommunications has indeed been staggering. Even some mobile telephones can now send and receive real-time video and yet the mobile telephone has only been in general use since 1991. In the investigations and news reports of the London bombings (July 2005) the use of mobile telephone photographs and videos brought both useful crime scene evidence and public insight into the atrocities of the incidents.

The immense increase in the number of households accessing the Internet can in some part be due to the development of Broadband (ADSL – Asymmetrical Digital Subscriber Line. Mode of digital transmission for exploiting existing old copper-cable networks in need of higher capacity in one direction than in the other, e.g. video-on-demand). Many users employ their computer to voice link to friends and family across the world without additional telephone cost over and above their ADSL subscription. This will have a significant impact on the telecommunications industry and in the long term is likely to reduce the cost of normal telephone calls.

In health care, a major breakthrough for the acceptance of telemedicine was during the first Gulf War (1991) where diagnosis and medical procedures at the front line were supported by experts from anywhere in the world. According to Carmichael (2005):

> It took the mission to Somalia in 1993 – a dangerous engagement that severely limited the military's ability to bring in medical supplies and staff – to prove that the tactic could be useful. There, military doctors used telemedicine mainly for treating eye wounds and broken bones: X-ray images and high-definition digital photographs were e-mailed to colleagues at Walter Reed.

The article includes information about the use of telepsychiatry and tele-counselling, both of which appear to have been extremely successful in meeting the needs of the military and the medics. We are aware that the most significant cost in health care is that of employee salaries, some hospitals have made great inroads in reducing these costs through outsourcing areas such as radiology. Most western hospitals use digital radiology today, and once a file is created it can be sent and viewed anywhere in the world, no longer does a hospital need to pay for a consultant radiologist to be on call locally. The image file is sent to the outsource, studied, report transcribed and file returned in a matter of minutes. Thus reducing waiting time for the patient and for differential diagnosis.

A recent survey carried out from the United States (Grady & Schlachta-Fairchild, 2005) on telenursing roles found that 'Survey respondents believe that currently the demand for telenurses is moderate, however a sharp increase in the demand is expected within three years.'

As we progress further into the twenty-first century it is likely that more and more use will be made of telehealth, for if we have achieved such successes in just over ten years, only our imagination will hold us back during the next ten.

Having given some thought to the overview of telehealth, we shall now consider four applications in more detail. The applications are in teletriage through the use of a nurse-led national call centre, telecare through the use of support infrastructure for carers in their own home, tele-patient education/support through mobile (cell) technology and tele-education through the delivery of a workshop across two continents.

## 7.2 Teletriage

The National Health Service (NHS) in England started a modernisation programme during the late 1990s which culminated in the NHS Plan (Department of Health, 2000). Within the programme a pilot nurse-led telephone call centre infrastructure was set up, first announced in the white paper, *The New NHS: Modern, Dependable* in December 1997. The infrastructure was extremely successful, and after the pilot which commenced in March 1998, in 2000, the service became an integral part of the NHS in England and Wales; the service is called NHS Direct and has since been enhanced with NHS Direct On-line and NHS Direct Digital Television. Scotland has since set up a similar service in 2002.

The objectives for the service were to

1. Offer the public a confidential, reliable and consistent source of professional advice on healthcare, 24 hours a day, so that they can manage many of their problems at home or know where to turn to for appropriate care;

2. provide simple and speedy access to a comprehensive and up to date range of health and related information;

3. help improve quality, increase cost-effectiveness and reduce unnecessary demands on other NHS services by providing a more appropriate response to the needs of the public; and

4. allow professionals to develop their role in enabling patients to be partners in self-care, and help them to focus on those patients for whom their skills are most needed. (Munro, et al., 2001)

The concept behind NHS Direct is that of either being an initial point of call for the public concerned about a current health issue they have and/or acting as a health resource to the public through information being made available either following a request or, in the light of general interest, such as MRSA (methicillin-resistant *Staphylococcus aureus*). The change process required was a move away from individuals visiting their community doctor or the emergency department for health issues that could be treated at home, thus releasing the community and hospital services for more serious ailments and pro-active care put in its most simple form. However, NHS Direct has had a significant impact on the more serious ailments and has through national audits demonstrated that it can save lives even at the end of a telephone line.

Sims (2002) raises an interesting point about the users of NHS Direct; he calls many of them the 'worried well' and muses where these individuals would have gone in the past for their information and health care access – possibly NHS Direct has replaced the over-the-wall conversation or the elders of an extended family now that very few walls exist and families are geographically separated. Sims goes on to comment: 'There is some evidence that NHS Direct does not curb demand on the NHS but allows the more appropriate use of health services that access it.'

This may be the key to the continuing use, development and extension of the service, better use of the services offered to the public, better information to the public and better clinical effectiveness to those in greatest need. NHS Direct operates using a series of evidence-based protocols. A person telephones the service and is connected to a trained operator who takes their details and ailment. Using the protocol pathway the caller is asked a series of questions the answers to which determine the direction taken in the pathway. At the end of the 'consultation' one of three outcomes are most commonly determined, either self care, professional care or emergency care. Some pathways are quite extensive whereas others, especially those where emergency care is the outcome tend to be extremely quick and to the point. If emergency care is required, the caller is informed that an ambulance is on its way – NHS Direct will alert the ambulance service during the call – and the operator will remain on line with the caller until the ambulance arrives.

If professional care is the outcome, the caller will be directed to their nearest health centre with the appropriate services to meet their needs. It is this added-value approach to the concept of a call centre that has held NHS Direct above other such telephone response systems. There are many anecdotal tales of difficulties with call centres, where the caller becomes frustrated with the responses received; this can be especially true when the centre is outsourced to perhaps another country. NHS Direct call centres have overcome this through having access to local information for anywhere in the country, so if a call is taken from another region, the caller can be given local information including public transport information as well as community doctor surgery opening hours, contact details etc. With the telephone network available in the United Kingdom, it is possible for the use of one telephone number to be routed to the 'local' call centre, if that is busy, the call can be re-routed to the next available call centre without any additional input by the caller. Without this infrastructure call-centre opportunities would be difficult to achieve. Thus, if professional intervention is required, the caller can be directed easily and quickly. Where a community practice is known by the caller, where the caller is registered, NHS Direct has an option to inform the practice of the call with the permission of the caller. This helps in preparing the practice for their intervention.

The Department of Health, the Welsh Assembly Government and the central management team of NHS Direct have identified a series of performance measures and service targets (Department of Health, 2000); these include the following:

- 90 per cent of telephone calls will be answered within 30 seconds (following the message)

- 90 per cent of symptomatic calls will be triaged within 20 minutes

- 90 percent of health information calls will be actioned or assessed within 3 hours

- Under 5 per cent abandonment rate (after 30 seconds and following the message)

- Under 0.1 per cent of all calls will receive the engaged tone

- Maintain at least 95 per cent of callers satisfied or very satisfied within the telephone service

  Additional targets in England

- 90 per cent of online enquiries will be responded to within 5 days of receipt

- Maintain at least 65 per cent awareness of the telephone service

Supporting the front-line telephone call centres are information officers who respond to on-line queries and to enquiries received as part of a call. Here, information from selected sources will be gathered and forwarded to the enquirer either by post, email or telephone. Thus NHS Direct performs yet another service to the population through education and information sharing.

NHS Direct is a 24-hour, 7-days-a-week service, as such it is available for callers who may just want to talk. In the early days of the service it was noted that many elderly people living on their own tended to call for a chat and where possible this service continues to be available today. A recent audit through the Commission for Health Improvement (CHI, 2003) stated:

> CHI was impressed with the way call handlers respect the dignity and confidentiality of service users. Sites are implementing the national confidentiality policy and training staff in accordance with this, and confidentiality is actively maintained across sites. Members of the public, service users and voluntary organisations said they value the helpline and advice offered by the service. They also found the advice given to be helpful and reassuring.

It would be wrong to imagine that the piloting, implementation and continued development of NHS Direct has been plain sailing and accepted by all; there have been many critics, mainly coming from health care professionals themselves. Another area for comment was the cost of such a triage national network:

> in March 2000 the average cost of a call to NHS Direct between January and March 2000 (£15.11) was higher than one published cost estimate of £8.00 per call (Hansard House of commons, 2000). Even in the long run, if sites are experiencing economies of scale, an optimistic estimate of the cost per call is still £3 higher at £11.10. (Munro, et al., 2001)

Interestingly, exact costing has ceased to be tabled in later reports about the service. Each time NHS Direct has expanded into sectors such as out-of-doors doctor's, pharmacies and non-urgent ambulances there have been concerns by the sector. This type of response is only to be expected, but over time both the service and the sectors have learnt from each other and now provide a better outcome for the public through working together. NHS Direct has its rivals in some areas, particularly that of information giving; a new website patient.co.uk claimed in May 2005 (e-Health Insider, 2005) to have received slightly more hits at 1.2 million in the previous month than NHS Direct On-line. There will be more such sites as the demand for knowledge continues, but in all NHS Direct needs to be thought of an integrated service made up of a number of elements of which information giving is one. It is the integration that could only be achieved through government support both in terms of finances and policy and NHS Direct has such support. This complex and increasing vital service within the NHS family is likely to grow and become more familiar with the public over the next five to ten years. As an example of teletriage there is nothing of comparable complexity available, and it must not be forgotten that it remains a service maintained by nurses.

## 7.3 Telecare

There are some who are concerned about the possibility of care becoming a 'robotic' experience for both the patient and carer. Maybe on some planets in a galaxy far away this is the case, but it is not yet true in this world. There are of course smart homes where sets of sensors are used to quickly identify where professional assistance maybe required, the sensors being part of system with acceptable parameters set and when these parameters are exceeded an alarm is raised. There are also systems where electronic tags are used to maintain surveillance on individuals who may wander and harm themselves, but these may not be the best examples of using technology to support care in the community.

The example for description here is different; it is about supporting carers in their own homes whilst they look after a relative or friend. The example for description is based upon a European funded project called ACTION (Assisting Carers using Telematics Intervention to meet Older persons Needs) (EU FP4 Action, 1994–1998) which commenced in January 1997 and was formed through collaboration between nurses in the United Kingdom, Sweden, Portugal, Eire and Northern Ireland. The primary aim was to 'maintain or enhance the autonomy, independence and quality of life for frail older and disabled people and their family carers, by using telematic technology – a combination of telecommunication and computer technology' (Magnusson, et al., 1998).

The project team was aware of the growing numbers of elderly in the population and was cognoscent of their wishes to remain at home for as long as was possible. In addition, there was understanding of the potential isolation felt by both the elderly person and their main carer. All of these issues were addressed by the project, and even though the project finished in 2000, further work is continuing as outlined by Magnusson (Magnusson & Hanson, 2004).

The project used the television as the delivery mechanism for the content and video links; sadly digital television was not available at the time, so a computer had to be attached and hidden as much as was possible from view. All control of the content was done using a handheld remote control unit in order to reduce the intrusion of using either an input device or keyboard.

Following extensive focus group discussions, questionnaires and literature reviews, individuals and organisations were identified to take part in the project in each of the countries; these consisted of nursing homes, hospitals, health care centres, social services centre and 20 family carers' homes. During the research it became clear there were five key areas which carers would find beneficial, these were identified as

**Caring in Daily Life** – consisted of three parts, transfer (moving) and handling, caring for people with incontinence and emergency situations.

**Planning Ahead** – supported the family carer in planning for the future regarding their caring situation.

**Break from Caring** – consisted of information describing various available respite care facilities.

**Claims and Benefits** – aimed at supporting the family carer with information about the different economic support available.

**Being a Carer** – consisted of a coping assessment section that focused on how family carers manage their caring situations and a coping strategies section aimed to help the family carer to develop a range of coping skills. (Magnusson, et al., 2002)

In addition, there was a help section and video capabilities through ISDN2b. The video link was available, again through remote control access, to the carers' local health centre, hospital and other carers with their permission as well as that of the project team; indeed I regularly received video calls from those participating whilst they were having a coffee break – it was clear from such informal access that the technology provided no fear to the users! During the project over 1,800 individuals impacted with the system, of these 767 were family carers; 249 cared-for persons and 786 were professional carers. Most found the system easy to use with all areas rating above 50 (mean) 60 (median) and helpfulness rated the highest (Sherwan, et al., 2000).

Each area was developed within the partnership and was available in the home language of those using the system. Three support areas were particularly important to the project partners; these were according to Magnusson (Magnusson, et al., 2002):

1. to reduce a sense of isolation;

2. to create a sense of presence;

3. to provide easier access to care professionals.

All of these support areas were directed towards allowing the individual and their carer(s) to remain at home for longer periods, respite care was available at any time and was taken by some, but others commented (Magnusson, et al., 2002, p. 373).

> It helps me personally because it's contact. It lets me know that I'm not on my own, whereas before you forgot there are other people who perhaps are in the same situation ... it gives me a wee bit of confidence and a wee bit more self-esteem in realising that the job you are doing is recognised. (Family carer, Northern Ireland)
>
> The videophone is useful because I don't feel so alone ... I have the videophone in case I need to contact someone. (Family carer, Portugal)
>
> The videophone is good. Better than an ordinary telephone. It's good to see each other. The person becomes more alive. You can see gestures. It's quite a change when you see the person you speak to. (Family carer, Sweden)

Maybe the ACTION Project has identified that users will use systems when they find benefit in the system, here was a case when use was found and the system was extremely well used. In the intervening years there has been considerable growth in the use of 'smart' technology, where a monitoring device is installed in an individual's home which has set parameters either side of which an alarm is raised. There is growing interest in building a supportive techno-logical network using the 'soft' humanistic areas tested in the ACTION Project alongside the emerging smart technologies. Care must be applied when using smart technology, an anecdotal story might be a useful reminder of difficulties. The story goes that an elderly gentleman with reduced urinary efficiency agreed to have a smart monitor fitted to his toilet system. The monitor would count the number of 'flushes' and would give out an alert to the local practice if these rose to more than 5 an hour. All was well until one afternoon the alert was sounded, the monitor recording over 20 flushes in a hour. A nurse was dis-patched to investigate. Upon arrival at the gentleman's house, she found he was entertaining about 30 of his friends to celebrate an anniversary. He was quite well and the nurse enjoyed a piece of sponge cake. Suffice to say, we are still learning about the use of smart technology.

So it came as a surprise when in July 2005, the Department of Health in England released a policy paper entitled Building Telecare in England (Department of Health, 2005). From April 2006, a grant of £80 million will be available for two years to support a change in the way in which care is supported for the increasing elderly population. According to the document the expected outcomes are as follows:

The grant should be used to increase the numbers of people who benefit from telecare, by at least 160,000 older people nationally. Its use will:

1. Reduce the need for residential/nursing care;

2. Unlock resources and redirect them elsewhere in the system;

3. Increase choice and independence for service users;

4. Reduce the burden placed on carers and provide them with more personal freedom;

5. Contribute to care and support for people with long term health conditions;

6. Reduce acute hospital admissions;

7. Reduce accidents and falls in the home;

8. Support hospital discharge and intermediate care;

9. Contribute to the development of a range of preventative services;

10. Help those who wish to die at home to do so with dignity. (pp. 6, 7)

All of the above is without doubt highly commendable, but is it achievable given the understanding of the technology by the majority of health and social care workers? It might appear to some that telecare is being seen as the new salvation to the ever increasing cost of health care and the anticipated demo-graphic changes especially in the increasing number of elderly people in western populations. Interestingly, the document does state that the finances available are not 'ring fenced' (this means funds can be applied for under the grant policy;

then if something more important arises, the money can be moved away from the application to meet the more important need) given that most NHS Hospital and Community Trusts are overspent (White, 2003) there must be a certain amount of cynicism as to how effective the new policy will be in reality.

Health care professionals need more experience with tele-technologies. One way of achieving this is through education, where technology can play a vital role and at the same time offer opportunity for professionals to use such technology in a safe and developmental environment.

## 7.4 Tele-patient education/support

We have been slow in the United Kingdom to harness mobile telephone technology, although in Europe we were early adopters of this technology through GSM (Global System for Mobile Communication). This was originally developed as a pan-European standard for digital mobile telephony; GSM has become the world's most widely used mobile system. It is used on the 900 MHz and 1800 MHz frequencies in Europe, Asia and Australia, and the MHz 1900 and 2100 frequency in North America and Latin America. Part of the reluctance to examine ways of use in health care was the public fear of brain tumours resulting from excessive use of mobile telephones (Coates, Hawks & Blair, 2005). These fears were concerned with the way in which mobile (cellular) telephones actually worked. In essence, GSM uses radio waves to transmit and receive data, the radio waves work within 'cells' of geographically mapped areas. If someone dials a mobile telephone, the radio waves are spread around the country in waves through these cells, rather like a ripple on a pond, first in a small area close to where the mobile telephone is registered, then wider a field until the recipient is found and the mobile telephone rings, or a message service interrupts in the case of not finding the mobile active. The ripple can extend across countries and across the world; for example, a user resident in the United Kingdom may be on holiday in continental Europe or Asia or Australasia, and if their mobile telephone is switched on it will ring and the call can be completed. A relatively cheap 'dual-band' (900 and 1800 GSM) mobile telephone can be used for these countries; a 'tri-band' (900, 1800 and either 1900 or 2100 GSM) is required if a user wants truly global coverage to include North and South America.

There was concern over these radio waves, particularly their strength at user level affecting the brain. However, further studies have demonstrated that there is no link between the use of mobile telephones and brain tumours (Frumkin, et al., 2001; Health Protection Agency, 2005), and now there are emerging trials using mobile telephones to support patient education, treatment and rehabilitation.

One such study by Professor R. S. H. Istepanian (UK-Principal Investigator) involves the development of a diabetes mobile management system between patients and diabetes specialists. The system is ubiquitous and integrates seamlessly with 3G Network protocols using intelligent PDA mobile terminals with Bluetooth wireless connectivity for measuring the blood and glucose levels.

The work is done in collaboration with Orange and Birmingham Heartlands Hospital NHS trust. As yet there are no results from the study available, but one thing is certain: moving to such technologies is bound to require changes in practice amongst health care practitioners.

Martin and Jones (2005) have gone some way into considering the implications to practitioners as we advance towards more reliance upon mobile information communication technologies (MICT) for clinical work practices in their review of selected pilot sites. In a table from their recently published article a number of issues arise (Table 7.1).

Are we ready in health care to trust something that has a limited battery-life? There are many anecdotes from friends and family which tell of forgetfulness in re-charging their mobile telephone and only remembering when they next need to use the device. What if a patient was as forgetful, and then missed a reminder to take a particular drug? HIV/AIDS sufferers who are supported through antiretroviral treatment need to take their drugs at a particular time; changes in the time can result in reduced effectiveness of the regime. It would be easy to think that reminders through mobile telephony could be the answer if a sufferer was travelling through time zones when mental calculation of the time is sometimes difficult. But what if the technology failed – where would responsibility lie? Further work needs to be initiated to reduce potential failure(s). The table reports well on knowledge-related issues and certainly there is increased use of mobile

**Table 7.1** Framework for analysing cases of MICT-in-use

| | | |
|---|---|---|
| *Technical and implementation issues*<br>Wireless technologies; privacy and security; battery life; training; hardware robustness | | |
| *Modalities of mobility*<br>Travelling–visiting–wandering; micromobility | | |
| *Possible effects of MICT on health care professionals' work practices* | | |
| Knowledge work related | Beneficial | Improved communication of care, collaboration and knowledge exchange. Removal of constraints for doing some tasks (e.g. prescribing, searching, evidence for decisions) |
| | Unclassified | Increased ability to send/receive information to/from the health care organisation. Effects on the nature/style of communication |
| | Undesirable | Easy access to (too much) data may bias, inhibit or slow decision making. Increased communication might not mean increased productivity |
| Time-space organisation | Beneficial | Reduced need for professionals' 'presence-related availability' to coordinate health care. New 'communities' might offer opportunities for continuities across time and space |
| | Unclassified | Increased rhythms of device use, of everyday life, of institutional change |
| | Undesirable | Disruption of boundaries between work and personal life. Intrusion on personal time and space |

*Source*: Reproduced with permission from Health Informatics Journal 11 (1) (c Sage Publications, 2005), by permission of Sage Publications Ltd.

devices such as portable palm-held storage. Where huge amounts of up-to-date information can be loaded and carried around in a small device, updates can be downloaded either wirelessly or through a base station allowing for synchronisation with the latest information quickly and effortlessly. Really all that is happening in this example is the transfer of text held within a book or on a website to a portable device, a mechanisation process rather than embracing the power of technology.

The table then addresses the issues of time and space and it is here that perhaps the real change will take place. Previous studies (Brennan, et al., 2001) have shown how the web can be used successfully in helping in the rehabilitation of patients following hospital intervention. It may be possible to harness mobile technologies to support rehabilitation programmes: at the time of writing I could find no such work in progress. With the increase in patient throughput (length of stay) in hospitals today it would seem that an effective rehabilitation process might reduce the potential of return admissions and/or reliance upon the stretched community services. A small study using telephone contact appears to be continuing the work started by Brennan (Hartford, 2005), the study appears to demonstrate that there is potential for extended work in this area and it is hoped that such work will take place soon.

We need to open our minds to the potential mobile telephony affords health care, but at the same time we must make sure that our rationale for use is sound, safe and has added value(s) to any process already employed. One way to improve our decision making is through use of the technology; perhaps one such use could be in our own education and training, which is discussed below.

## Tele-education

It has been said that part of the role of education is not only the development of new knowledge, but also the learning of that new knowledge within a safe environment (Siemens, 2003); with the increase in the development of telematics in health care, it is right and fitting that clinicians get to experience and understand the technology in a safe setting. Through use, clinicians may find themselves in a better position to find suitable care support which would benefit from telematics interventions.

An element of the environment includes those around us whilst we learn. Of course we can learn individually, but more frequently we learn in groups; this is common in formal courses offered at postgraduate level, and these groups can be single or multi-professional. More common still is the gathering of such learning groups in rooms within institutions for education. In these groups we exchange formal and informal ideas and knowledge, although from a diversity of backgrounds we share a common experience for a certain number of hours a week.

The evolution of learning at a distance brought about a significant change to the culture of learning (McIntosh, 2001). No longer were individuals grouped together in rooms, although a group might be formed, it tended to be people working at different levels and a different pace within an asynchronous forum, thus reducing the common support whilst going through the experience of learning (Dron, 2001). Generally, with such courses there would be intervals of group togetherness such as a summer school or study weeks/weekends (Joyes, Fisher & Coyle, 2002). These gave an opportunity to mix with others and share the common experience.

Since the late-1980s (Nagy, 2004) there has been a developing movement towards the use of technology to support learning at a distance. One of the early exponents of such learning was the English National Board's Computer Assisted Learning (ENB CAL) Project (Procter, 1991). This was within the domain of nursing and started in 1988. After three days together in a room, participants returned to their place of work, downloaded further material using a computer and network, then returned their assignments using the same network. In addition, all involved had access to discussion forums, where issues could be considered and addressed, with responses being available to all participants. Over 750 people took part during the three years of the project. Others followed, and now it would be inconceivable not to use the Internet and World Wide Web to support students at a distance.

Sadly, although the technology today is light years ahead of that used nearly twenty years ago, there is still considerable evidence of mechanised use rather than true use of the power the technology offers. Frequently we see lecture notes on the web, PowerPoint presentations and documents for students to access (Massy, 2002); this is using the web as a storage device, which is fine as long as it is recognised as such. But the technology can offer our students and us so much more, including direct access at appointed times to key figures in the content area – this would not be possible any other way without significant financial investment. The development of virtual learning environments has to some degree widened the horizon, but through informal observations it would appear that very few teachers use such powerful tools for much more than a text page-turner with a few web links and graphics.

It seems as though that to overcome the possible disadvantaging of students studying at a distance teachers using virtual learning environments write masses of text in an effort to demonstrate to the student that they are unlikely to miss anything as everything is written down. We know that in a face-to-face lecture a student is likely to retain around five per cent of the content delivered (Meister, 1998), we know that postgraduate students in particular are not fond of didactic teaching methods (Arseneau & Rodenburg, 2000) and we know that the most powerful way to assist learning is for the student to be able to internalise the content (Biggs, 1994). So why isn't this done using the technology? The response would appear to be that we are not sure how thus many different methods are being practised with varying acceptability results.

In one course with students in Canada on Health Informatics held in 2004, a new model was tried and appeared to work extremely well with the post graduate mature students. The model used an asset-based approach (Procter, 2005), with the tutor linking the assets through minimalist dialogue supported by selected assets of articles (copyright permission granted), video snippets, audio snippets, still images, quality assured web sites, PowerPoint presentations and anything else considered helpful. The course was divided into units, each unit taking two weeks to complete. In the first week, the students examined the assets and began to form opinions of the area under consideration. The second week was devoted to an online discussion where the assumed opinions and further knowledge could be exchanged. The course was driven by these discussions, for it was through these that the richness and diversity of the discussion came to the fore. The students met three times during the course – an introductory session, a communication session and an evaluation session. A description of the communication session now follows giving an example of the use of extended tele-education.

The session was to help students understand the roles and relationships involved with hierarchical management structures as found in health care organisations and the passage of information in order to achieve a given goal. Of course it would have been ideal to be with the students in person, but this was not possible due to time and cost constraints. This would be the first time the students and distance tutor had met over and above in discussion forums.

The workshop was run from Sheffield in the United Kingdom with a second tutor assisting at the Canadian site. In addition, expert help was available for the multiple video cameras at the distant site so that different angles could be seen; angle selection was in part directed from Sheffield through verbal instruction. The Sheffield tutor was shown throughout on a screen in the classroom. Following introductions, the students were given their roles and tasks, and the workshop commenced. With the advantage of multiple cameras at the distant site, it was very nearly as good as being present. After two hours, the workshop concluded with successful achievement of the required outcomes. The cost had been around £40 for the Internet protocol connection. Interestingly, when the link was disconnected at the Sheffield site there was a feeling of isolation felt by the tutor as the individual was no longer part of the group. The workshop was followed up by discussion amongst the group: included below are some of their comments:

**Student A:**

How did this game change how I view information systems and the information system that I use? Good question. I think it illustrates the flow of communication and the problems that can occur during the communication process. It also demonstrates the importance of objectivity and feedback, and the difficulties encountered when there are time restrictions that add stress to the process. I like the Collaborative Model presented in this weeks reading, and especially the comments made in the introduction.

Cheryl Lamb writes 'Technology should only play a supportive role ... it is the people and processes supported by appropriate technologies that deliver real results'. Perhaps we should be supporting the development of Decision Support Systems to deliver options when vision is difficult to translate and time is restricted. Or perhaps we should be careful not to let the human element get swept to the side in our pursuit of technology.

**Student B:**

It was this conclusion that put the icing on the cake. You gave me the key piece to a puzzle in life that I have been working on. Here are some ideas/lessons I have come up with (keeping in mind, this is now 20/20 vision – as M puts it). First, identify your resources. Most of us assume we have the same resources as others. How many times do errors from simple, inaccurate assumptions create some of the biggest problems? I fear I would have clued in too late to think of this one. Meanwhile, I wonder … do we need to see our staff as resources? Very viable ones, I might add. What simple assumptions do we make without really getting to know them?

**Student C:**

… the idea of having a teacher/student relationship feels quite natural must be attributed to the communications we have had in our discussion groups … so I see I am able to gain a sense of people through the medium.

Maybe the most interesting thing about the student's comments is that they appear to have taken the use of a video link to run their session as quite normal; indeed, two did not include it in their comments at all. There are many risks involved with moving away from teacher-led instruction to student-facilitated learning but in the experience of the author these are far outweighed by the growth of knowledge and challenge in questions of the students. The richness and diversity that adds so much to the learning process has been brought into the course by the students, which is how it should be as they are the ones currently in practice; and with a little guidance and knowledge support through the assets and teacher interaction in the discussion forums it is a highly rewarding method of teaching. Tele-education is still in its pioneering phase, but the world is becoming smaller and there is a significant likelihood that education through video and web will increase to meet demands.

## 7.5 Final reflection

In this chapter we have explored the uses of telematics in health care; four particular areas where nursing can demonstrate a lead have been described further. There are an ever increasing number of 'tele' developments; some will be of great success and some will be of questionable effectiveness, like the pen that could write in space which allegedly NASA spent around $2 million developing whereas the Russians used lead pencils with equal effect.

Given that our brief trawl across telematics started with dermatology – not a very convincing application in the long term – it maybe appropriate to end with a message that is around professionalism versus using technology for technology's sake. If telematics is useful to all parties then it should be used; if not then alternatives should be employed.

### LEARNING ACTIVITIES

1. Telematics is an accepted word which includes many different technology applications. Individually can you list two applications by name and describe them? Then in your group, discuss the identified applications and make a list of the best six applications with their brief descriptions.

2. The essence of tele-health is that it is health care at a distance. In your group, consider and write a list of the educational requirements for health care professionals to ensure safe practice using this technology?

3. Tele-health is not a cheap way to deliver health care. There are those who would argue that in urban areas the use of tele-health is null and void as people can easily get to see a health care practitioner. With another person discuss this claim and determine whether or not tele-health should be available in urban as well as rural areas. Write down both sides of the argument and report them to the group.

## References

Arseneau, R. & Rodenburg, D. (2000). The Developmental Perspective. In Pratt, D. & Associates (eds), *Five Perspectives in Adult and Higher Education.* Florida, FL: Krieger Publishing Company.Barlow, J., Bayer, S. & Curry, R. (2005). Flexible homes, flexible care, inflexible organisations? The Role of Telecare in Supporting Independence. *Housing Studies, 20*(3), 441–456.

Biggs, J. (1994). Student Learning Research and Theory – where do we currently stand? In Gibbs, G. (ed.) *Improving Student Learning – Theory and Practice.* Oxford: Oxford Centre for Staff Development.

Brennan, P. F., Moore, S. M., Bjornsdottir, G., Jones, J., Visovsky, C. & Rogers, M. (2001). Heartcare: An Internet-based information and support system for patient home recovery after coronary artery bypass graft (CABG) surgery, *Journal of Advanced Nursing 35*(5), 699–708.

Carmichael, M. (2005) Combat stress teams and telemedicine: The new strategies for helping soldiers cope with war. *Frontline*, http://www.pbs.org/wgbh/pages/frontline/shows/heart/readings/telemedicine.html [Accessed 28 May 2005].

Coates, S., Hawks, N. & Blair, A. (2005). Mobile phones tumour risk to young children. *The Times Online*, 12 January.

Commission for Health Improvement (CHI). (2003). *NHS Direct 4 Years On*, London, CHI Publication.

Department of Health. (2000). *The NHS Plan: A Plan for Investment, a Plan for Reform.* London, HMSO.

Department of Health. (2005). *Building Telecare in England.* London, HMSO.

Dron, J. N. (2001). Achieving self-organisation in network-based learning environments. PhD Thesis. University of Brighton, UK.

E-Health Insider. (2005). Patient information site rivals NHS Direct Online. *E-Health Media Ltd*, No 173, 12 May.

EU FP4 ACTION (TAP-DE-3001) (1994–1998). *Project Fact Sheet.* http://www.cordis.;u/src/g_021_en.htm [Accessed 3 June 2005].

Frumkin, H., Jacobson, A., Gansler, T. & Thun, M. J. (2001). Environmental carcinogens – Cellular phones and risk of brain tumors, *CA Cancer J Clinics, 51*, 137–141.

Grady, J., & Schlachta-Fairchild, L. (2005). The 2004 international telenursing role survey. *Executive Summary*, iTelehealth Inc and Mt Aloysius College.

Hansard House of Commons. (2000). *Column 269WH*, 6 April, UK, Westminster Hall.

Hartford, K. (2005). Telenursing and patients' recovery from bypass surgery. *Journal of Advanced Nursing, 50*(5), 459–468.

Health Protection Agency. (2005). *Mobile Telephony and Health*. http://www.hpa.org.uk/radiation/ understand/information_sheets/mobile_telephony/ index.htm [Accessed 20 September 2005].

Joyes, G., Fisher, T. & Coyle, D. (2002). Developments in generative learning using a collaborative learning environment. In Banks, S., Goodyear, P., Hodgson, V. & McConnell, D. *Networked Learning 2002: A Research Based Conference on e-learning in Higher Education and Lifelong Learning*. Sheffield. University of Sheffield.

Magnusson, L., Berthold, H., Chambers, M., Brito, L., Emery, D. & Daly, T. (1998). Using telematics with older people: the ACTION project. *Nursing Standard, 13*(5), 36–40.

Magnusson, L., Hanson, E., Brito, L., Berthold, H., Chambers, M. & Daly, T. (2002). Supporting family carers through the use of information and communication technology–The EU project ACTION. *International Journal of Nursing Studies, 39*(4), 369–381.

Magnusson, L. & Hanson, E. (2004). Working with older people and their carers to research and develop responsive ICT support services. *Health Informatics Journal, 10*(1), 83–88.

Martin, H. M. G. & Jones, M. R. (2005). What's so different about mobile information communication technologies (MICTs) for clinical work practices? A review of selected pilot studies. *Health Informatics Journal, 11*(2), 123–134.

Massy, J. (2002). Quality and eLearning in Europe survey report 2002. *Training Foundation*. http://www.trainingfoundation.com/research/default.asp?PageID=798 [Accessed 11 April 2005].

McIntosh, M. (2001). *Sustainability & Innovation, Learning and Cultural Change*, The Sigma Project, Warwick Business School, University of Warwick.

Meister, J. C. (1998). *Corporate universities: Lessons in Building a World-class Work Force* (rev. edn.). New York: McGraw-Hill.

Mouratidis, H., Manson, G. & Philp, I. (2003). Analysis and design of the eSAP: An integrated health and social care information system. *Health Informatics Journal, 9*(2), 89–92, Sage Publications.

Munro, J., Nicholl, J., O'Cathain, A., Knowles, E., & Morgan, A. (2001). *Evaluation of NHS Direct First Wave Sites: Final Report of the Phase 1 Research*. The University of Sheffield, UK.

Nagy, A. (2004). *E-Learning, E-Content Report 6 an Integrating Report by ACTeN Anticipating Content Technology Need*. EU IST Publication, p. 5.

National Statistics Omnibus Survey (NSOS). (2005). *Individuals Accessing the Internet: Access to Internet from Home*. Family Expenditure Survey (April 1998–March 2001); Expenditure and Food Survey (April 2001 onwards).

Procter, P. (1991). Use of a National/International telecommunications network for distance learning in an adult environment. In Hovenga, E. J. S., Hannah, K. J., McCormick, K. A. & Ronald, J. S. (eds), *Nursing Informatics 91* (pp. 710–720), Amsterdam: Springer-Verlag.

Procter, P. M. (2005). An asset based model for online learning. (Unpublished).

Scholes, M., Bryant, Y., & Barber, B. (eds) (1982). *The Impact of Computers on Nursing*. B.V, North Holland: Elsevier Science Publishers.

Sherwan, J., Tetley, J., Clarke, A. & Hanson, E. (2000). Evaluation of the outcome of the project, the telematics applications and technical system in relation to user friendliness, user acceptance and quality and function of the technology which have been adapted, developed and used. Unpublished EU Project Report DE3001, Brussels. Sims, P. (2002). Correspondance – NHS direct and new paradigm of medical care. *Journal of Public Health Medicine, 24*(1), 70.

Siemens, G. (2003). Learning ecology, communities, and networks extending the classroom. *Elearnspace*, http://www.elearnspace.org/Articles/learning_communities.htm [Accessed 11 April 2005].

Thompson, T. G. (2004). Administration's efforts to increase the use of information technology throughout the health care industry. *Statement before the House of Representatives Committee on Energy and Commerce, Subcommittee on Health*. 22 July 2004. http://www.hhs.gov/asl/testify/t040722.html [Accessed 2 August 2005].

White, C. (2003). One in seven NHS trusts facing 'significant' financial difficulties. *British Medical Journal, 3*, 326–680.

---

### RECOMMENDED READING

Debnath, D. (2004). Activity analysis of telemedicine in the UK. *Postgraduate Medical Journal*, 80, 335–338.

Finch, T., Mort, M., May, C. & Mair, F. (2005). Telecare: Perspectives on the changing role of patients and citizens. *Journal of Telemedicine and Telecare*, 11, Supplement 1, 51–53.

Hartford, K. (2005). Telenursing and patients' recovery from bypass surgery. *Journal of Advanced Nursing*, 50(5), 459–468.

UK Telemedicine and E-Health Information Service: http://www.teis.nhs.uk/

# Computer Utilisation in Patient Care Systems

Jacqueline Lopez-Devine and Rose Sherman

## LEARNING OBJECTIVES

When you have read this chapter, you will be able to:

■ Discuss the primary reasons why health care organisations are moving towards the adoption of computer utilisation in their Patient Care Systems.

■ Describe the Information System's Life Cycle and why nursing involvement in each phase is the key to the successful utilisation of automated patient care systems.

■ Identify the lessons learned from a case study presented from a practice setting where point of care technology was introduced.

■ Discuss Everett Rogers' adoption of Innovation Theory as a useful framework to consider in overcoming staff resistance to the adoption of computer utilisation.

■ Identify best practices, professional practice issues and future implications for nursing with the introduction of computer utilisation into existing patient care systems.

## KEY WORDS

■ computerised order entry

■ electronic medical record

■ health information technology

- information systems life cycle

- nursing informatics

- patient care systems

## 8.1  Computer utilisation in patient care systems

When compared to the progress made in other industries, health care has been slow to adopt computerised technology into patient care systems (Larkin, 2005). The nursing profession began to use computers in patient care settings in the 1970s (Saba & McCormick, 2001). Initial computerised patient care systems were piecemealed together and lacked integration and interfacing capabilities with other organisational systems. The lack of integrated patient care systems meant clinicians were forced to search several data sources for patient information resulting in increased workloads and slowed information retrieval (Barrett, 2000). In the mid-1980s, nursing informatics, computer utilisation and patient care systems began to take a more organised approach as the concepts of systems and data integration and interfacing became more prevalent among the main vendors supplying these automated systems (Johnson, 2003). By the mid-1990s, the health care informatics industry began re-evaluating and redesigning computerised applications for patient care systems to assure they were appropriately integrated into the clinical process. It also later began to provide clinicians a multitude of hardware options designed to facilitate clinical practice (Rivers, Blake & Lindgren, 2003). Today's nurse is more technologically savvy than the nurse of the past. This growing interest in technology by nurses accompanied by improvements in computer hardware and the use of increasingly integrated systems have accelerated the adoption of computerised patient systems. In addition, the introduction of new roles related to nursing informatics has also helped to ease the transition in nurses' adoption of computerised systems.

This chapter focuses on computer utilisation in patient care systems. The discussion includes the primary reasons why health care organisations are utilising computer systems, the implications of the information system life cycle, lessons learned from a case study, the potential value of applying Everett Roger's adoption of Innovation Theory as a framework to overcome staff resistance, an overview of the nursing research, best practices in computer applications and some of the current and future issues for nursing.

### Driving forces for computer utilisation

The health care industry trends towards 'managed care, downsizing ... consolidation' and the existing nursing shortage have provided health care organisations with a strong impetus to reduce operating costs, and utilise integrated systems in patient care systems (Barrett, 2000). Integrated computer systems that speak to each other not only facilitate the job of the end user and reduce duplication in data entry but also reduce the probability of medical errors. Integrated systems aide health care organisations in obtaining their goals of becoming paperless and moving towards a completely electronic medical record. Current problems with paper patient care records include the following:

▪ non-integrated data collection;

▪ data redundancies;

▪ difficult-to-access information. (Barrett, 2000)

These problems can be avoided with carefully designed electronic medical records. Well-designed patient care systems used simultaneously with user-friendly hardware lead to a successfully implemented electronic medical record. Special attention needs to be taken to carefully select the right type of hardware to meet the needs of specific clinical settings. Today's health care organisations acknowledge that a well-designed and implemented clinical information system not only facilitates an EMR but also 'eliminates duplicate tasks, helps nurses reduce errors, and keeps documentation to a minimum' (Meadows, 2002). Early involvement of end-users in the selection, design and implementation of patient care systems means participation of the end-user in the 'information systems life cycle' (Craig, 2002). The nurses' involvement in the 'information systems life cycle' is the key to successful prolonged utilisation of a new auto-mated patient care system. The same is relevant for the selection of hardware used in the clinical setting.

## The information systems life cycle

The information systems life cycle is a continuum. The continuum includes (1) The system planning phase; (2) the analysis and design phase; (3) the imple-mentation phase; and (4) the support phase (Ball, et al., 1995). The entire cycle involves a process that is structured in order to assist in the development of a clear plan. It includes the upfront definition of the end users requirements and 'every day' functionality needs. This is particularly important in patient care systems where the designers of the computerised system may have no clinical experience. The cycle works successfully when meaningful input is solicited from active stakeholders. The process of system selection and design needs to be driven by the end users. If a hospital is selecting a new system for electronic nursing documentation, involving staff nurses who use the current documen-tation system is important to avoid problems with newly designed systems. Nursing informatics specialists have emerged as a key group to provide organ-isational support through all phases of the information systems life cycle. Nursing leaders are now recognising that their involvement in the selection, design and implementation of computerised systems in nursing care areas is a critical success factor (Cato, 2005).

## Computer utilisation: A Case Study

Palms West Hospital, in Loxahatchee, Florida, is a 175 bed community hospital offering a full range of clinical services. The hospital is part of the Hospital Corporation of America (HCA). HCA is composed of locally managed facilities with over 190 hospitals and 82 outpatient surgery centres in 23 states, England and Switzerland. In 2000, 126 employees and physicians within the Healthcare Corporation of America met to present ideas that eventually assisted in the development of a new medication safety initiative known as an electronic medication administration system (eMAR) which included medication and patient armband bar coding. HCA worked with the vendor company Medical Information Technology, Inc or, more commonly known as MEDITECH, to develop the initiative. MEDITECH is a software vendor in the health care informatics industry that provides integrated solutions for hospitals, ambulatory care centres, physicians' offices, long-term care and behavioural health facilities and home health organisations.

The system is designed so that each patient admitted to an HCA facility receives an armband with a bar code. The bar code corresponds to the patient's current medical record, including drug history, allergies and laboratory results. Bar code identifiers also appear on plastic shrink-wrapped doses of medication. Before a medication is administered, bar codes on the patient armband and the medication are scanned, allowing the nurse or therapist to verify that the right patient is receiving the right drug in the right dose at the right time. The software checks each medication against the patient's drug history and laboratory results. If conflicts or potential drug interactions are identified, warnings alert the nurse to double check, verify and/or call the doctor before administering the medication.

Palms West Hospital utilised the information systems life cycle in the implementation of the electronic medication administration record. During the system-planning phase, the Chief Nurse Officer (CNO) selected a system planning team to assist with the decision-making process of key policy related issues. The team consisted of various members from stakeholder departments and disciplines involved in the medication administration process with nursing and pharmacy as major participants in the process. Though the hospital did not need to select a vendor for the product, it did need to design how the hospital would utilise the electronic medication administration record and bar code system. The CNO defined the scope, objective and timelines of the project to the planning team. A projected 'go live' date was selected and presented to the team.

Once the team was clear on the mission, the information systems project manager assisted the team through the analysis and design phase. The team surveyed the units to assess the current practice of medication administration through out the hospital. Issues and problems in the current system were identified. The experiences of other organisations were also analysed. Best practices in medication administration were defined and developed into policy to support the new system. The team met regularly to ensure timelines were followed and they played a role in the selection of hardware. After research and comparison, the team selected a compact mobile medication cart that had on top of it a physically secured laptop. The mobile cart connected to the hospital network through the use of wireless technology.

The project manager and CNO both played key roles in leading the team through the design phase. The team had the responsibility of determining the best solutions to identified requirements through the use of the new system. Decisions such as whether to include intravenous fluid solutions such as normal saline and dextrose in the eMAR and bar coding were analysed by the team.

Once most of the system requirements were defined, the eMAR system was designed and built. The implementation phase then began to take shape. Key trainers were selected by nurse managers to become system experts or super-users at the point of care. A train the trainer approach was used with the super user group. The trainers attended a four-hour class on the use of the eMAR system. The system planning team opted to pilot the project on a 43 bed Medical/Surgical Unit. The super users trained all the Medical/Surgical Unit's staff during the first two weeks of the 'go live' schedule. Every two weeks after the Medical/Surgical Unit went live, another in-patient nursing unit would 'go live' with the new eMAR and bar coding system. The total implementation time to role out the project to all inpatient areas was approximately three months.

## Lessons learned

Palms West Hospital is currently in the support phase of the eMAR system. Issues such as replacement of laptop batteries and proposed new improvements to hardware are being addressed. The key to proper system support is a shared departmental responsibility between Information Systems and Nursing. Nursing needs to report issues that need follow-up in a timely manner while the Information Systems department is accountable for ensuring that changes are quickly made to the system as problems and issues occur. Nurse Managers continue to discuss eMAR and bar coding implementation and educational concerns with staff at meetings. These issues and concerns are shared regularly with the CNO at team leadership meetings. Effective communication ensures that common concerns are filtered up for appropriate resolution. Palms West Hospital through the use of teamwork, change management and informatics is moving forward in preparing their nurses for the future. Although during the initial transition more time was spent in medication administration, properly designed point of care clinical documentation systems, automated medication administration systems, physician order entry systems and online clinical data repository, the systems should ultimately allow nurses to spend more time on critical nursing tasks versus documentation. Key success factors in this implementation project included CNO support and involvement of staff at the point of care in decisions about how the system would be implemented and a well-executed implementation and staff education plan. To date, 119 HCA hospitals are using the eMAR and bar coding system (HCA 2005). In December 2004 alone, eMAR at HCA hospitals evaluated 7.4 million medication doses. The bar coding system noted 233,540 warnings and prevented 183,215 doses from being administered. Without eMAR, HCA anticipates 2 per cent of doses would be given in error. HCA's results with eMAR have been instrumental in encouraging the FDA to develop a standardised bar code system for use throughout the pharmaceutical industry and at all hospitals to reduce the risk of medication errors that can seriously harm patients (HCA, 2005).

It is imperative to develop strategies that promote change based on an understanding of the behavioural aspects of change and the human decision-making process. Conrick and Ribbons in Chapter 9 note that 'implementing an information system … is a major organisational change process'. To this end, Everett Rogers' Adoption of Innovation Theory (Rogers, 1995) provides a useful framework for identifying the human response patterns of change. The framework can provide guidance to nurse leaders at all levels when implementing computerised patient care systems into nursing practice.

## 8.2   Everett Rogers' adoption of innovation theory

A nurse's daily practice involves gathering data from assessments, monitoring equipment, communicating with patients and the patient's medical record. The nurse interprets data, organises it and turns it into information about his or her patient's care and condition. The information may be used to generate new knowledge about his or her patient's condition or to intervene on the person's behalf. Although computer utilisation and properly designed patient care systems are keys to helping nurses manage data efficiently and effectively, as outlined by Barnard in Chapter 1, the introduction of new computerised systems brings about changes in each nurse's daily practice.

Promoting computer utilisation and implementation of patient care systems requires intense planning and education to prepare the end users both technologically and psychologically. The psychological components involved are process oriented, dealing with human factors that facilitate or inhibit change (Hilz, 2000). The technological preparation is task oriented, with implementation broken down into step-by-step phases that are focused and manageable. It is essential to stress that process and task are closely intertwined during planning and implementation of patient care systems as both technological and psychological aspects must be considered for a successful implementation.

Rogers (1995) uses a set of categories entitled 'adopter categories' to reflect the inherent differences between individuals with regards to their rate of adopting an innovation such as implementation of a patient care system. It is essential to familiarise oneself with these categories in order to facilitate moving a group towards adoption of a new process. There are five categories: innovators; early adopters; early majority; late majority; and laggards (Hilz, 2000).

Innovators are venturesome and eager to try new ideas; they are usually very useful as members of a steering committee. The early adopters are very integrated into the social structure of the target group; they are the role models and usually the first to 'buy into' an innovation. They make excellent troubleshooters during the system implementation and are often used by organisations as trainers or super users at the point of care. The early majority adopts new ideas just before the average individual does; they are not considered leaders but are followers of the early adopter group. This group can be persuaded either individually or through the early adopter group. The late majority are the sceptics and they require intense communication. It should be understood that positive results may be delayed with this group. The laggards are the very last to adopt an innovation; they distrust change. The most effective means of dealing with this group is to try and determine the source of their resistance in order to negotiate their support for the process of implementing change.

Another consideration when implementing change in an organisation is the five stages of the decision-making process, otherwise, known as Rogers' Innovation–Decision Process (Hilz, 2000). They are knowledge, persuasion, decision, implementation and confirmation. Certain behaviours are present in each stage, and it is important that you recognise them in order to effectively influence change. Knowledge is information gained when the nurse is exposed to the innovation; it is crucial that the change agent reinforce the need for change during this stage. Persuasion is the attitude (favourable or unfavourable) that the nurse develops towards the innovation. During this stage, the key stakeholder should provide the end users with information. A decision regarding the proposed innovation occurs when the nurse partakes in activities which influence the choice to accept or reject the innovation. During the decision stage, managers should provide technical assistance and guidance to the end users. Confirmation of a decision occurs when the nurse seeks reinforcement of the decision that has been made. During the confirmation stage, leadership should provide encouragement to the end users. This will ensure that end-users provide creative improvement ideas about the new innovation.

The Palms West Hospital success story cited in the case study earlier incorporated all aspects of Rogers' Innovation-Decision Process. Key nursing leaders and stakeholders recognised the importance of Rogers' five adopter categories through out the system planning, analysis and design, implementation and support phases of the EMAR project. Understanding innovation theory and using strategies such as those recommended by Rogers to counterbalance resistance enable nurse leaders to promote technology changes that hold great promise for the future of nursing and health care.

## 8.3 Best practices in computer applications in patient care systems

Technology can be effectively used in health care to improve processes, standards and protocols that result in better patient outcomes and enhanced patient safety. The electronic medication bar-code technology described in the case study earlier, which was originally pioneered in late-1990s by the Department of Veterans Affairs and later implemented in 168 of its medical centres, has had significant impact in the reduction of medication errors (Case, Mowry & Welebob, 2002). This technology is part of a broader technology called auto-identification. Radio-frequency identification (RFID) or bar-code capability can automatically identify a person or item. The technology will soon be used to mark surgical sites to reduce the number of wrong side surgeries and in the future patients may have implantable chips with their medical histories encoded in them (Taylor, 2005). Examples of other computer applications currently being implemented in health care environments that impact nursing practices include the following:

1. paperless electronic medical records;

2. computerised physician order entry;

3. electronic intensive care units;

4. smart intravenous delivery pumps;

5. personal digital assistants.

### Paperless electronic medical records

The terms electronic health record (EHR) and electronic medical record (EMR) are sometimes used interchangeably but there are distinct differences between the two. The EMR is maintained by a health care agency or in a physician's office and contains all clinical documentation of care, health histories, laboratory results and medication history. In contrast, the EHR contains more general patient information usually in a summary format and can be considered to be a subset of the EMR (Orlovsky, 2005). At this time worldwide, most medical records are still stored on paper. In the United States, only 20–25 per cent of hospitals have adopted paperless electronic medical records and many of these systems do not include computerised order entry (Hillestad, et al., 2005).

Despite the slow adoption of the electronic medical record, the advantages of computerised medical records in the health care environment are becoming evident to organisations who embrace them. Timely access to patient records can avoid the costly duplication of tests. It has been estimated that as much as 1/3 of the 1.8 trillion dollars that the United States spends on health care could be avoided if the collection and organisation of medical records was online (Frist, 2005). Another significant area of communication confusion in current paper medical records involves the interpretation of handwriting. This problem is eliminated with the typed entry of notes and orders.

Well-designed electronic medical records can also provide alert prompts to nurses to ask questions ranging from allergy history to the patient risk of falls. It has been suggested that with the availability of alert prompts, a compelling reason for nursing professionals to embrace the EMR is that it has the potential to improve both the consistency and quality of nursing care by reminding nurses of key areas where data needs to be collected.

EMRs can be linked with other technology tools used in health care agencies such as medication administration systems, IV pumps and vital sign monitors. The data can be automatically downloaded into the EMR avoiding documentation duplication. From a nursing perspective, having all the information about the patient in a centralised place available to multiple interdisciplinary team members at the same time decreases the frustration of looking for the missing pieces in medical records.

The transition to EMRs in some health care organisations has prompted concern that more nursing time is spent documenting when these new systems are implemented. The introduction of new electronic documentation systems may initially result in more time spent documenting but research suggests that the time is not excessive (Korst, et al., 2003). The ability of an electronic medical record to improve patient safety and clinical quality may relieve the anxiety of nurses and enable them to provide safe, better care which has a positive impact on job satisfaction and outcomes.

## Computerised physician order entry

Improving the safe delivery of medications is vitally important to nursing professionals (Smith, 2004). In the United States, organisations such as the Leapfrog group and the Institute of Medicine have strongly advocated the adoption of computerised physician order entry (CPOE) as a significant strategy to reduce medical errors. The Department of Veterans Affairs, the largest integrated health system in the United States with 170 medical centres and 800 outpatient clinics, has fully implemented computerised order entry and now estimates that they have more than 1.3 billion orders online (Department of Veterans Affairs, 2005). Despite national discussion, progress has been slow and only about 5 per cent of US health care organisations have adopted CPOE (Cato, 2005). The irony that fast food restaurants employ technology to process their orders in a computer while most health care agencies currently do not is not lost on either consumers or health care professionals (Dunbar, 2004).

The implementation of computerised physician order entry has the potential for a transformational impact on nursing practice. CPOE is a system that allows health care providers to enter orders into the computer. The orders are sent electronically to hospital departments, the hospital pharmacy and the nursing unit where the patient has been admitted. For nurses, the computerised entry of orders eliminates the frustration of reading poor handwriting and calls to clarify orders with physicians. Turnaround time to receive medications is reduced because pharmacies directly receive orders. Error prescribing prevention software is built into the system to notify physicians of problems with drug dosages and incompatibilities. CPOE has been shown to reduce serious prescribing errors in hospitals by more than 50 per cent (Leapfrog Group, 2005).

## Electronic intensive care units

The care of patients in intensive care units is extremely complex. Recent research has suggested that when the care of patients in critical units is managed by specially trained physicians called intensivists, patient care outcomes are improved (Breslow, et al., 2004; Leapfrog, 2005). Shortages of these specially trained physicians have led to the development of a new technology called electronic intensive care units or eICUs. An eICU is an electronically monitored intensive care unit that enables physicians, nurses and other health care team members from a remote location to immediately access expert advice and consultation on their patients. The settings resemble the operations in an air traffic control tower (Nowlin, 2004).

Using voice, video and data software and hardware, the remote intensive care unit staff can monitor heart rates, blood pressures and oxygen saturations of patients in the eICUs under their management (Nowlin, 2004). They can also check ventilator settings, review x-rays and laboratory reports and care plans that are transferred electronically. Through video cameras, they can interact with patients, their families and staff and even zoom in close enough to check pupils. The eICU is designed to provide another set of watchful eyes with highly seasoned intensive care unit staff and the opportunity for immediate consultation in critical situations. The software used in eICUs is sensitive enough to detect trends and subtle changes that nurses and doctors at the bedside might miss.

Health First is a hospital system that implemented an eICU in 2004 in south-eastern Florida to enhance intensive care unit coverage across three hospitals (Wood, 2005). Although initially concerned about invasion of privacy issues, nurses now find that there are strong reasons to embrace the trend. Having expert staff immediately available for consultation is comforting to both staff and patients. The remote staff uses a doorbell to announce themselves to both staff and patients before the camera is turned on in the room. The smart alerts in the eICU systems monitor for changes in physiological signs that might indicate a deterioration in condition. Early studies conducted at Health First and other health care systems that have implemented eICUs have demonstrated a decrease in length of stay and reduction in mortality of intensive care unit patients (Coye, 2005; Smith, 2005).

### Smart intravenous delivery pumps

Medication errors are a serious concern in today's health care environment. Over 60 per cent of the most serious, preventable adverse drug events are IV-related (Smaling & Holt, 2005). Manual programming of infusion devices is one of the most common causes of IV medication errors (Brown, 2005). Smart IV pumps have embedded software with clinical algorithms that store dosage levels for various medications and alert for possible errors in drug administration. There are fewer programming decisions for nurses to make averting the potential for error. Facilities can also customise dosage limits around their patient population making them especially useful in paediatric settings.

Data is continuously collected and in some cases downloaded into EMRs. The information collected is allowing health care organisations to monitor their intravenous medication practices and capture both actual and potential adverse event information (Steingass, 2004). A challenge for nurse leaders in environments that utilise smart pumps is the monitoring and assessment of all the data that is available from these pumps.

### Personal digital assistants

Mobile computing using personal digital assistants (PDAs) are a growing technology in health care environments. Data capture and retrieval using a PDA by physicians, nurses and allied health care professionals, are enhancing patient care and improving efficiency. Handheld computers, both Palm and the Pocket PC, currently are being used for e-prescribing, charge capture, research, reference, patient education, accessing daily schedules and as clinical tools. The PDA has been embraced by nurse educators as an important part of the academic toolbox and is now required in some academic nursing programmes.

In most settings at the present time, nurses are using PDAs as a reference tool to look up medications, calculate drug dosages, review policies and procedures. In the future, PDAs will be Internet connected in a wireless environment to EMRs and other technology devices. Charting in the future may be done on the PDA with periodic downloads to a desktop computer. This technology and interconnection will be particularly important in home health and visiting nurse situations where access to information is needed to deliver the best care. The PDA holds great promise to revolutionise nursing care. In the future, much of the information that nurses need to care for patients will be available in their pockets with these handheld devices.

## 8.4 Nursing research on computer utilisation

Initial nursing research on computer utilisation in nursing practice focused on the themes of cost-effectiveness, cost-benefit ratios, subjective evaluation by the nurse end user and the effect nurses' attitudes had on the adoption of computer technology. The preliminary research done was largely subjective and lacked consistent statistical testing needed to verify the reliability and validity of findings.

Both the field of Nursing and Informatics need to address existing gaps in continuing education opportunities for nurses that are practicing today. It is imperative that clinicians stay on top of the latest health care technology as well as understand the application of constant changes occurring in this area especially since change is not always appropriate and developments must be supported with evidence. Technology-related topics is the most rapidly-growing area of continuing education for nurses but gaps remain in many nursing curricula with respect to developing skills and knowledge for critical evaluation and efficient application of technology for quality care. Many remain ill-equipped to prepare students for an increasingly automated health care environment.

Staggers, Gassert and Curran (2001) defined four levels of informatics competencies for practicing nurses. Further analysis should focus on how nurses' informatics competency affects the implementation of a clinical information system. For example, once clinical informatics specialists have this type of data, they can work with nursing educators to help develop informatics curricula in nursing schools and health care facilities. Wood (2005) explored the relation between student nurse's computer competency and their success in passing the United States RN-NCLEX (National Council Licensing Examination), which is now computerised. It was found that students comfortable with computer technology felt they performed better on their nursing license exam.

A point of strong debate in the literature is the impact of computer utilisation on work processes and staff time. McLane (2005) studied the perceptions of nursing staff prior to the introduction of an electronic medical record. She found staff were generally positive but had concerns that it would increase their workload and the confidentiality of patients would be more difficult to protect.

Smith, et al., (2005) evaluated the impact of computerised charting on staff attitudes, completeness of documentation and time spent charting. Their study found that although staff attitudes about computerised documentation were negative, the completeness of their documentation improved and time spent in documenting did not increase.

Moody, et al., (2005) in their research evaluated the needs, preferences and perceptions of nurses associated with the EHR that was being used in their facility. The nurses reported that they felt confident with their skills but over half used a duplicate method of documentation because it was inconvenient to use the EHR at the bedside. Room size, slow computers and inadequate access to computers affected preferences and usage. The majority of nurses in their study agreed that the EHR was a help to care and improved documentation. Studies such as these assist software vendors in developing new systems that meet the needs of the end user and are evidence based. Importantly, there is sufficient evidence as to the actual effects of this type of care. Further studies need to be done to analyse the impact of newer clinical information systems on clinical practice and care delivery.

**Professional practice issues**

Despite the rapid development of technology designed to enhance patient care, the application of these technologies in patient care systems are not without challenges. For the first time in professional practice settings, there are four generations in the workplace with different experience levels and comfort zones with technology as it is introduced. The youngest nurses in the workforce sometimes called millenniums grew up in a digital age and are restless with the slow pace of technology adoption in health care. In contrast, the oldest generation of nurses still employed often called the veterans grew up without computers and computer literacy is a skill that they have had to develop over time (Case, Mowry & Welebob, 2002). Educators are challenged to incorporate technology into nursing education yet caution about the need to help students understand what to do when technology fails. In the future, the use of technology in organisations may be a key difference in the recruitment and retention of younger staff. New graduates who have worked with computers throughout their lives will look for organisations with cutting edge technology (Cato, 2005).

Nursing leaders are recognising that involving staff in the selection, implementation and evaluation of technology is critical to insure that appropriate technology is adapted to the workflow in a productive manner with good patient outcomes. Taylor (2005) notes that basic health information goals must be addressed when computer applications are evaluated and these include

1. informing clinical practice;

2. interconnecting clinicians;

3. personalising care;

4. improving population health.

Successful implementation means tracking the unintended consequences that a change in technology will bring. Changes to skills and knowledge in clinical practice and information security of health care information are examples of issues that are challenging in an electronic environment. When medical records are handwritten and stored in hospital charts or file rooms, they are accessed by very few health care professionals. EMRs in contrast provide broad access to information and protection of patient privacy has become extremely difficult (Harman, 2005). In 1996, the United States Congress enacted the Health Insurance Portability and Accountability Act (HIPAA). A requirement of this act was the development of privacy rules governing the use of EMRs (Flores & Dodier, 2005). HIPAA and additional privacy rules that have been enacted in the United States have led to the application of sophisticated technologies designed to control access to information.

Health care facilities have spent enormous financial resources to establish identification and authentication systems for authorised individuals to access information in the EMR along with the establishment of audit trails (Harman, 2005). Nurse leaders have recognised the potential for broad access to patient information and the need to establish a culture of confidentiality within our workforce (Calloway & Venegas, 2002).

## 8.5 Final reflection: Future implications

The potential impact of technology on the future of the health care industry is enormous. Roger's (1995) Adoption of Innovation Theory presents a useful framework for introducing new technology into organisations. The case study outlined in this chapter is an example of a best practice in the introduction of technology. New computer applications that are already being implemented in some settings include paperless electronic medical records, computerised order entry, electronic intensive care units, smart IV pumps and personal digital assistants.

A challenge for nurses worldwide is to balance the value of new technology with patient outcomes and care costs in health care environments struggling with financial pressure, regulatory requirements and workforce shortages (Smith, 2004). Building appropriate technology infrastructures in the health care industry requires massive financial investment and professional change. Debate rages about who should pay for it (Larkin, 2005) and reimbursement for technology investments continues to be a major policy issue. With a reduced worldwide nursing workforce, the potential of technological advances to improve patient safety and facilitate the work of nurses through robotics or other means needs to be explored.

Technology has the potential to improve access to health care globally and to be a great equaliser for countries which historically have had limited access to cutting edge treatments from clinically expert staff. The type of technology used in electronic intensive care units can provide real time consultation in care from clinical experts to health care staff who are thousands of miles apart. The nursing profession has the opportunity to take a pivotal role in ensuring that computer applications in patient care systems are used to help correct the historical inequalities of access to care globally (Simpson, 2002).

A first step towards the future is for nurses to embrace the potential of information technology and become involved with decisions in their organisations about its use. The world has entered a digital age and technology will play a significant role in the future of health care. Technology can sometimes have unintended consequences on practice both positive and negative. The impact of technology on professional nursing practice will require ongoing nursing research to help guide the decisions of nurse leaders about the implementation of computer utilisation in patient care systems.

## LEARNING ACTIVITIES

1. The idea for medication bar-coding originally came from a nurse who questioned why foods in grocery stores were bar-coded and not medications. In small groups, discuss a computer application technology that you have seen used outside of health care that could be applied to patient care systems.

2. In small groups debate the issue of who should have access to a patient's electronic medical record and under what circumstances?

3. As a group, list strategies for computer applications in patient care systems that could be initiated to improve health on a global level and reduce health care disparity.

## References

Ball, M. J., Simborg, D. W., Albright, J. W. & Douglas, J. V. (1995). *Healthcare Information Management Systems: A Practical Guide.* New York: Springer-Verlag.

Barrett, M. J. (2000). *The Evolving Computerized Medical Record.* [Retrieved 3 September 2005] http://www.health-informatics.com/issues/2000/05_00/barrett.htm

Breslow, M. J., Rosenfeld, B. A., Doerfler, M., Burke, G., Yates, G., Stone, D. J., et al. (2004). Effect of a multiple-site intensive care unit telemedicine program on clinical and economic outcomes: An alternative paradigm for intensivist staffing. *Critical Care Medicine, 32*(1), 31–38.

Brown, B. (2005). Optimize IV infusion safety. *IT Solutions Nursing Management Supplement, 36*(10), 19–22.

Calloway, S. D. & Venegas, L. M. (2002). The new HIPPA law on privacy and confidentiality. *Nursing Administration Quarterly, 24*(4), 40–54.

Case, J., Mowry, M. & Welebob, E. (2002). *The Nursing Shortage: Can Technology Help?* (1 Health reports). California: First Consulting Group for the California Healthcare Foundation.

Cato, J. (2005). Winning support for a clinical information solution that meets nurses' needs. *Nurse Leader, 3*(1), 42–45.

Coye, M. J. (2005). *The eICU and New Business Models in Health Care.* [Retrieved 10 October 2005] http://www.ardsil.com/cgi-bin/ubbcgi/ultimatebb.cgi?ubb=get_topic&f=28& t=000006

Craig, J. B. (2002). The life cycle of a health information system. In. Englebardt, S. P. & Nelson, R. (eds), *Healthcare informatics: An interdisciplinary approach*. St Louis, MI: CV Mosby, pp. 181–208.

Department of Veterans Affairs. (2005). *What We Accomplished in Healthcare, Benefits and Memorial Affairs*. [Retrieved 10 October 2005] Department of Veterans Affairs Web Site: http://www.1.va.gov/health_benefits

Dunbar, C. N. (4 October 2004). *Safety First – Writing's On the Wall*. [Retrieved 10 October 2005] http://community.nursingspectrum.com/MagazineArticles/article.cfm?AID=12902

Flores, J. A. & Dodier, A. (2005). HIPAA: Past and future implications for nursing. *Online Journal of Issues in Nursing*, 10(2), [Retrieved 9 October 2005] www.nursingworld.org/ojn/topic27/tpc27_4htm

Frist, W. H. (2005). Why We Must Invest in Electronic Medical Records. *San Francisco Chronicle*, (25 July). p. 7.

Harman, L. (2005). HIPAA: A few years later. *Online Journal of Issues in Nursing*, 10(2), [Retrieved 9 October 2005] www.nursingworld.org/ojn/topic27/tpc27_2htm

Hillestad, R., Bigelow, J., Bower, A., Girosi, F., Meili, R., Scoville, R., et al. (2005). Can electronic medical record systems transform health care: Potential health benefits, savings and costs. *Health Affairs*, 24(9), 1103–1117.

Hilz, L. M. (2000). The informatics nurse specialist as a change agent: Application of innovation-diffusion theory. *Computers in Nursing*, 17(6), 272–281.

Hospital Corporation Of America (HCA). (2005). *EMAR and Bar Coding*. [Retrieved 13 October 2005] http://www.hcahealthcare.com/CPM/HCAMedicationSafetyInitiativeFactSheet.pdf

Johnson, R. I. (2003). *Health Care Technology: A History of Clinical Care Innovation Health Care Technology Project 1*. [Retrieved 29 August 2005] http:www.hctproject.com/content/pdf/hct1_wp_Johnson.pdf

Korst, L. M., Eusbeio-Angejac, A. C., Chamorro, T., Aydin, C. E. & Gregory, K. D. (2003). Nursing documentation time during implementation of an electronic medical record. *Journal of Nursing Administration*, 33(1), 24–30.

Larkin, Howard (2005). Uncle Sam wants your EHR. *Hospitals and Health Networks*, 78(2), 38–53.

Leapfrog Group. (2005). Management Systems: A Practical Guide. *The Leapfrog Group Fact Sheet*. [Retrieved 10 October 2005], http://www.leapfroggroup.org/about_us/leapfrog-factsheet. New York: Springer-Verlag.

McLane, S. (2005). Designing the EMR planning process based on staff attitudes toward and opinions about computers in healthcare. *CIN: Computers, Informatics, Nursing*, 23(2), 85–92.

Meadows, G. (2002). The nursing shortage: Can information technology help? *Nursing Economics*, 20(1), 46–48.

Moody, L., Slocumb, E., Berg, B. & Jackson, D. (2005). Electronic health records documentation in nursing: Nurse perceptions, attitudes and preferences. *CIN: Computers, Informatics, Nursing*, 22(6), 337–344.

Nowlin, A. (1 October 2004). *Get Ready for the Virtual ICU*. [Retrieved 10 October 2005] http://rnweb.com/rnweb/article/articleDetail.jsp?id=114162

Orlovsky, C. (2005). The endless nursing benefits of electronic medical records. [Retrieved 9 October 2005] http://www.nursezone.com/job/DevicesandTechnology.asp?articleID=1427

Rivers, F. H., Blake, C. R. & Lindgren, K. S. (2003). Essentials of computers for nurses: Informatics for the new millennium. *Online Journal of Nursing Informatics*, 7(3). [Retrieved 29 August 2005] http:eaa-knowledge.com/ojni/ni/7 database

Rogers, E. (1995). *Diffusion of Innovations*. New York: Free Press.

Saba, K. A. & McCormick, K. A. (2001). *Essentials of Computers for Nurses: Informatics for the New Millennium*. (3rd edn.). New York: McGraw-Hill.

Simpson, R. (2002). No-borders nursing. How technology heals global ills. *Nursing Administration Quarterly*, 28(1), 55–59.

Smaling, J. & Holt, M. A. (2005). Integration and automation transform medication safety. [Retrieved 10 October 2005] http://www.healthmtgtech.com/archives/0405/0405integration_automation.htm

Smith, C. (2004). New technology continues to invade healthcare. What are the strategic implications/outcomes. *Nursing Administration Quarterly, 28*(2), 92–98.

Smith, K., Smith, V., Krugman, M. & Oman, K. (2005). Evaluating the impact of computerized clinical documentation. *CIN: Computer, Informatics, Nursing, 23*(2), 132–148.

Smith, L. (2005). Close watch at a distance for critical care patients. *Washington Post* (30 January). p. C04.

Staggers, N., Gassert, C. A. & Curran, C. (2001). Informatics competencies for nurses at four levels of practice. *Journal of Nursing Education, 40*(7), 303–316.

Steingass, S. K. (2004). Preventing harm with high risk medications. Presentation at the meeting of the *American Society of Health System Pharmacists*. (8 December), Orlando, FL.

Taylor, N. T. (2005). National Health IT coordinator applauds nurses as 'early adopters'. *IT Solutions Nursing Management Supplement, 36*(10), 2–6.

Wood, R. M. (2005). Student computer competence and the NCLEX-RN examination: strategies for success. *CIN: Computers, Informatics, Nursing, 23*(5), 237–240.

## RECOMMENDED READING

American Nurses Association. (2001). *The Scope and Standards of Nursing Informatics Practice.* Washington, DC: American Nurses Publishing.

Hunt, E. C., Sproat, S. B. & Kitzmiller, R. (2004). *The Nursing informatics Implementation Guide.* New York: Springer-Varlag.

Saba, V. K. & McCormick, K. A. (2001). *Essentials of Computers for Nurses.* New York: McGraw-Hill.

Thede, L. Q. (2003). *Informatics and Nursing.* Philadelphia, PA: Lippincott, Williams & Wilkins.

# Informatics, Information and Nursing: A Critical Examination

Moya Conrick and Bob Ribbons

---

## LEARNING OBJECTIVES

When you have read this chapter, you will be able to:

- List the potential benefits of information technology to nursing practice.

- Provide a pragmatic view of the limitations of information technology in nursing.

- Discuss the interplay of information, politics and organisational change and how these elements might impact nursing.

- Discuss the role of clinical decision support in the provision of improved patient care.

---

## KEY WORDS

- change

- clinical decision support

- information systems

- nursing informatics

- politics of informatics

---

## 9.1   Nursing and information technology

Information Technology (IT) refers to all forms of technology used to create, store, exchange and use data, information and knowledge (McKeown, 2001). Essentially IT provides the infrastructure for a networked economy and has become a highly pervasive and ubiquitous component of modern society. It is hard to imagine a bank, an airline or grocery shopping without interacting with information technology; it is taken for granted and is expected. In many respects, IT has made life easier and more convenient while arguably making our lives more complex. Consider the impact on the workplace where we are inundated with information, much of it superfluous, but all of it requiring some form of attention.

The use of computers and information technology to support the management of health information is also becoming more ubiquitous and has been the impetus for the rapid evolution of nursing and health informatics in the past few years. Information systems can store unlimited data for administrative areas and can track the patient throughout a hospital stay and across geographical boundaries thanks to advances in standards and interoperability (Conrick, 2006a).

The use of information technology in health has also changed the models of health care and the manner in which health care workers deliver patient care. Every day nurses deal with huge volumes of patient care information, at every stage of the care delivery process. They are engaged in data collection and analysis, problem solving, clinical judgement, decision making, documentation and communication. There is nothing new about this. What has changed is the acuity of patients/clients in need of health care and a subsequent exponential growth in the volume and complexity of health care data. An overlay of health IT has the potential to make our information handling either more efficient or significantly more complex.

Proctor (2000) has suggested a humanistic information model in which the key elements of acquisition, processing, storage and dissemination of information are seen as a set of interlocking cogs. Each cog has an independent function. However, no one cog can act independently of the others to which it is connected (Proctor, 2000). This approach is a departure from the traditional linear process model and more accurately describes the complexity of clinical information. An intrinsic aspect of this model and its metaphorical reference to cogs is that the turning of cogs simultaneously generates and transfers power. The subsequent power is directly proportional to the value placed upon the information being processed (Proctor, 2000). Given this proposition, the need to determine the value for nursing information becomes apparent.

Health Informatics (HI) is a socio-technical and scientific discipline that deals with the collection, storage, retrieval, communication and optimal use of health related data, information and knowledge. The discipline uses the methods and technologies of the information sciences for the purposes of problem-solving and decision-making thus assuring quality health care in all basic and applied areas of biomedical sciences for the community it serves (Health Informatics Society of Australia, HISA, 1998). There are many branches of Health Informatics and Nursing Informatics is one of these.

## Nursing Informatics

Nursing informatics (NI) has had a somewhat difficult beginning and although it has been recognised as a nursing specialty for the last two decades many nurses do not understand the essence of this discipline. The definitions of NI have changed over time to reflect the developments in nursing practice and technologies. The most widely accepted definition comes from the International Medical Informatics Association – Nursing Informatics (IMIA–NI) group who redefined NI in 1998 as '... the integration of nursing, its information, and information management with information processing and communication technology, to support the health of people world-wide.'

In their various roles and specialty areas, nurses handle large volumes of data and NI is concerned with all aspects of this. For example, it encompasses all aspects of access, retrieval and efficient use data, information and knowledge to support decision-making, which in turn enhances the quality, effectiveness and efficiency of nursing care. While information and communications technology is essential to nursing practice to support the development and disseminate new knowledge, they can also support and empower clients' decision-making and health care choices (Conrick, 2005).

NI offers a range of tools that assist in advancing nursing as a professional research-based discipline (Saba, 2001). Large databases enable the timely collection, storage and analysis of vast amounts of data. This is made available and retrievable as information in a manner that nurses require it to support their practice. It also allows nurses to critically review their practices based on evidence provided by these systems. This is significant as Sim, Sanders and McDonald (2002) estimate that currently only around twenty per cent of clinical practices are underpinned by research. They see this as partly due to the impediments of illegibility, fragmentation and lack of standardisation of nursing data that paper records impose on researchers and the establishment of evidence-based practice.

While the tools of information management offer to improve the collection, management, processing and communication of nursing data, their uptake by the nursing profession is significantly impeded by numerous factors (Englebardt & Nelson, 2002). This includes education, language and the paternalistic treatment of nursing or exclusion of the profession by some decision makers. Simpson (2004) also discusses technophobia or the fear of technology that nurses reportedly have towards IT. He also discusses the thought that technology might replace the nurse's position and sees these issues as further impeding nursing uptake of technology. However, Kirkley and Stein (2004) may be closer to the mark finding that nurses resist the introduction of technology because the benefits of technology take time to occur and all they see is technology adding to their already busy schedules.

Nurses are often asked to use information systems that are foreign to them and often have limited appreciation of its power and potential to support their practice (Conrick, 2006b). St Joseph Hospital in America, however, was able to demonstrate tangible positive outcomes for example, 'reduced time spent on paper charting by 50 per cent with the implementation of online documentation releasing 1.5 hours in a 12 hour shift to focus on patient care' (Kirkley & Stein, 2004, p. 218). Historically, nurses have embraced technology when it assists their work and provides improvements in patients' outcomes. They must be encouraged to join the NI debate, to use new technology and to overcome any fears, uncertainty and wariness of change. Barriers must be recognised and discussed, benefits made clear, and long-term results for improved delivery of quality care communicated to minimise sources of technology resistance (Kirkley & Stein, 2004).

## 9.2 The potential benefits of information technology

The potential of information systems to produce beneficial outcomes in health care are well documented (Chu, 2001; Lipp & Williams, 2000; Protti, 2005; Silver, 2002). The digital collection of data afforded by information technology overcomes the limitations of paper records and enhances nurses ability to access relative, accurate and organised information to continually evaluate and effectively improve nursing practices (Bakken, Cimino & Hripcsak, 2004; Conrick, et al., 2006c). The traditional paper-based record only provides a third of the data that a clinician needs to provide adequate patient care (Anderson, 1999). Unlike paper-based systems, automated systems provide multiple, simultaneous access to information in a distributed format. Information systems also allow the user to view information in a variety of formats depending on their requirements. The clinician is able to customise the way in which information is displayed by sorting, graphing or tabulating data. This ability to manipulate clinical data can also yield significant benefits in terms of clinical research.

IT is seen as facilitating best practice both in its potential to streamline health care and reduce adverse events. IT can be used in clinical areas to reduce the time spent documenting patient care and provides more accurate information by eliminating inaccuracies and data redundancy (Herlihy & Allen, 2005; Huges, 2000). In traditional paper-based information systems, data items such as a patient allergy need to be entered multiple times on multiple forms. It only takes one instance where this duplication is overlooked to potentially result in an adverse event. Computerised information systems on the other hand, enable the automatic, multiple use of this data, eliminating manual duplication and ensuring critical information is available at all times.

Nurses are freed from clerical duties, theoretically to devote more time to patient care due to the introduction of greater efficiencies and reductions in the need for duplication. In one example, Morrissey describes the introduction of an electronic medical record and reports a reduction of 2.75 hours in the time nurses spent on administering medications. This represented a cost saving of AUS$2.4 million in nursing time which was reallocated away from manual documentation and back to direct patient care (Cox, 2003).

IT enhances the timeliness of health data communication, providing optimal access to the best possible information on which to base clinical decisions (Huges, 2000). The almost instantaneous communication afforded by these systems ensures that information in a useable format is in the right place at the right time. This significantly improves the continuity of care across health care services, reduces the duplication of investigations, clinical errors and inefficient administrative processes (Reinecke, 2005).

The need to achieve increasing levels of quality in care delivery whilst realising resource efficiencies (i.e. cost effective care) has resulted in the development of specialist information systems (Van de Velde & Degoulet, 2003). Anderson (1999) suggests that the successful implementation of these systems will heavily depend on integrating data from a variety of sources. Integrating clinical data from multiple sources such as laboratory, radiology, pharmacy and those captured at point of care, either manually or downloaded directly from physiologic monitors is the basis of robust clinical tools such as decision support systems and automated clinical pathways.

Clinical decision support systems, inherent in many clinical systems, act to safeguard the patient and the clinician, enhancing safe practice. Automated clinical pathways and system alerts ensure that therapeutic measures are not overlooked. Collection of clinical data at the bedside is not only accurate; it leads to more accurate clinical decisions. The integration of evidence-based practice guidelines and policies into information systems provides a rich knowledgebase and when it is based on evidence ensures that 'best practice' becomes an integral part of clinical care.

## 9.3 The politics of information access

Undoubtedly, nursing faces a plethora of opportunities and challenges in the future. Many of these will come from increasing demands for improvements in quality and cost-effective care and will emanate from government, society and our colleagues in other health disciplines. Nursing must be able to address these issues within the context of an increasingly information-intensive environment. Whilst information systems can support more informed decision-making, their use also impacts on existing power and political relationships.

The old adage that 'information is power' has certainly proved true over the years. The implication of whoever possesses information holds some degree of control is, of course, based on the assumption that the information held is of value to someone else. There is a counter saying; 'information is power but to share information is more powerful' and historically this has been the situation in nursing. Reflect a moment on a typical ward situation in which nurses' act as information conduits, receiving information from one source and subsequently relaying it to its intended recipient. As an information broker, nurses have enjoyed a certain degree of power.

Nonetheless, it is in the dissemination of this information that others come to see the influential role nurses play in health care. This is a key element; after all, there is not much point in holding information if no one else knows you possess it. This information brokerage phenomenon has conferred a certain level of power and influence on nurses relative to other health-related disciplines.

However, there are implications for this relationship where IT provides access to clinical information in a distributed fashion and it is possible that the traditional dependency that other health disciplines have had on nursing will change. Borthwick and Galbally (2001) suggest contemporary nursing suffers from a weakness in self-concept and consequently, a reduction in political status and empowerment. If this is real, the loss of nursing's clinical gate-keeping role with its inherent power and influence could have far-reaching implications for the profession. These authors also note nursing faces a number of tensions between different conceptions of its role and status and its relationship to other health service disciplines. It is in the area of information management that these tensions are, arguably, most evident.

## 9.4 Information, politics and organisational change in a technological environment

The last decade has seen a transformation of work practices and an explosion in information technology systems. This has been supported by substantial investment in the information management infrastructure in the health sector because of a belief that technology will improve patient care and deliver quality, cost effective health outcomes. It also stems from a realisation that the computer can offer health greater flexibility, reduced paperwork, greater access to information and a reduction in time spent by clinicians performing non-clinical tasks (Conrick, et al., 2004).

However process design, technology acquisition and implementation must be interwoven, it is not as simple as buy-and-install. Accordingly, Saunders (in PricewaterhouseCoopers LLP, 2005, p. 28) sees it as '… a hand-in-glove thing … technology can only be as good as the process'. Digital integration into a setting requires the deployment and integration of a complex, connected series of technologies to create a smoothly running system that fully exploits the technology and empowers the health workforce to more effectively fulfil their responsibilities (PricewaterhouseCoopers LLP, 2005).

The digitalisation of hospitals entails major organisational transformations and substantial business risks that must be managed. Risks include cost overages and failure to gain expected returns on the investment made. Health is a rarity because few other industries spend huge amounts on IT while facing the risk that when the project goes live a significant proportion of staff will refuse to use it (PricewaterhouseCoopers LLP, 2005).

### Political impetus for informatics integration in health care

While most other information intensive industries, such as banking and insurance, have used IT for more than two decades, health care has been much slower. The Economist (2005), reports that the United States health care industry is spending only around two per cent of revenue on IT, compared with ten per cent in other information-intensive industries. Australian e-Health market figures are comparable to these findings (CHIK Services, 2004). Given Australia's aging population, all health care providers and levels of governments recognise the urgent need for capital investment in health IT infrastructure to reduce expenditure and improve the quality of patient outcomes.

In Australia, as in many other countries, Governments are at the forefront of implementations and are providing the impetus for accelerating the adoption of IT in health. Transforming health care process through technology can have a powerful impact on an organisation and nursing, as the single biggest provider of health services, has the capacity to 'make or break' these implementations.

Developing insights into the interaction of nursing information, politics and organisational change in contemporary IT environments is essential to the modern nursing environment. To achieve this, nurses need to develop specific skills in

1. leadership with preparation to engage in the political process;

2. change management;

3. determining the economic value of nursing information; and

4. designing and deploying information systems including electronic health record systems.

## Leadership and preparation to engage in political processes

The direction of health care in Australia is currently the focus of much political debate. The impetus is the concern over service demands and delivery to an aging population and the potential cost implications. The transience of our population, a volatile and mobile workforce and staff shortages, together with economic imperatives to increase efficiency and effectiveness are also of concern. Stakeholders agree that performance and improvements in the sector are both necessary and achievable but conditional upon the implementation of a more interconnected health system designed to support health reform (Boston Consulting Group, 2004).

The implementation of information systems is an important priority for health planners and managers as a key driver for performance improvement. Their introduction makes it possible to consider alternatives that reduce the bureaucratic management of health services while retaining planning, funding and accountability in government control. The aim is to combine market solutions such as competition with rational planning, public accountability and democratic control. It is here that nurses need to adopt a more politically savvy approach to their interactions within health care organisations.

The ability of policy makers to formulate health policy depends on health care information services to provide the data they need. This comes from the front line of health care but this is the very area in which data collection is the least developed. The need for information across health care is now being increasingly understood. Nursing can be guaranteed direct influence in the formulation of health policy if there is 'ground floor' nursing input to the development of information systems dedicated to this data collection.

At present, most health care organisations have information systems that are inadequate to meet future information needs, and they are often limited to specific functions. For example, an information system dedicated to billing alone has no capacity to integrate clinical outcomes and process of care with financial outcomes. Clearly, integration cannot be achieved within a single health care organisation; the chances of providing integrated health services across the state, let alone the nation, remain a rather distant dream. If nurses are to play any part in health policy development and for them to be heard by policy makers they must be empowered with information and skills in data analysis. All nurses have an extended role as stakeholders in health care planning and must assume this role.

### Nursing's contribution to change management

Information systems are tools to assist people working in complex health care environments. Implementing an information system is more than just solving technical issues. It is a major organisational change process. Health care organisations must justify their work output in financial and qualitative terms. To be successful, an information system should, ideally, repay its investment by providing managerial, operational or patient information that benefits the organisation in terms of improved decision making, ease of data transfer, understanding by all users and recipients and ultimately improved care.

Existing managerial, cultural and social aspects of the organisation as well as individual behaviour are likely to change with the availability of new information and its technology. To be useful, the implementation must also support specific issues in the organisation. In the absence of a pre-existing information culture, some individuals may be unused to handling information or using technology resulting in less effective use of new capabilities.

Some may see the system as a threat; while clinicians may be concerned it may distract them from their patient care role. In addition, restructuring may have to take place; such as the introduction of new departments to manage the information function and so change internal politics. An understanding of business process re-engineering and change management can position nursing in a valuable position to take advantage of these internal political changes.

### The need to determine the economic value of nursing information

Anderson (1999) discusses the need for high-level sponsors as a means of increasing acceptance of introducing clinical information systems. These high-level sponsors or clinical champions are often drawn from senior medical staff or from the hospital executive. Examples of senior nursing staff fulfilling this role are scarce in the literature. This may be more reflective of nursing's position in traditional health care political hierarchies and their ability to influence organisational decision-making rather than any ability to implement information systems!

Contemporary health care organisations are driven both politically and economically by those elements identified as revenue raisers. The areas within the organisation that can generate the greatest revenue tend to have a proportionally greater contribution to the organisation's decision-making process. In most organisations, however, nursing is described as a 'cost center' and not recognised as the unique resource that it is.

Inherent difficulties in quantifying the cost benefit of nursing's contribution to patient care have historically restricted its ability to exercise political power in health care. Tsuru and Yasuaki (2000) propose that information on which effective nursing care is based holds an inherent value that can be quantified, not just in terms of improved patient outcomes but in actual dollar values. If this is true, then nursing services, rather than being seen as a cost to health care organisations, actually generate revenue by providing effective care that reduces complications, lengths of stay, readmissions and subsequently, costs.

A recent study by Hall, Doran and Pink (2004) suggested a higher proportion of professional nurses were in the staff mix on medical and surgical units in Ontario teaching hospitals associated with lower rates of medication errors and wound infections, while Unruh and Byers (2002) noted a link between inadequate staffing and poorer patient outcomes. The latter study also point to research indicating that reductions in nursing staff and skill-mix generally have negative impacts on nursing staff and patient care.

### Design and deployment of information systems including electronic health record systems

It can be argued that more than any other factor, the technical aspects of information systems present the greatest challenge to nursing. Conversely, it also provides nurses with unparalleled opportunities for engaging in health care informatics.

The need for nurses to develop specific information systems design and deployment skills has been well articulated in the literature (Ball, 2001; Ball, et al., 2000; Hersher, 2000; McCartney, 2004). These authors argue that nurses possess a unique skill set that lends itself well to roles within health care informatics. Nurses possess excellent problem-solving skills and are adept at prioritising in critical situations whilst maintaining a global view of the issues involved. They demonstrate well-honed skills in data collection, documentation, analysis and evaluation and are renowned for leadership and people management skills. When combined in a technology environment, these skills make nurses excellent candidates for project managers and indeed nurses have been appointed to the Health*Connect* trials in this capacity.

## 9.5 Nursing informaticians

Currently, most nurses 'stumble' into informatics positions by being in the right place at the right time. The organisation may require a clinician for an informatics steering committee or someone to assist the rollout of a clinical system.

In these cases, the organisation may not be looking for an individual with extensive technical experience. Often individuals with strong computing backgrounds have difficulty in understanding clinical work practice flows which may hamper their ability to communicate effectively with clinicians. A nurse on the other hand, with some, albeit often limited computing experience, possesses the appropriate people management and communication skills to fulfil these roles effectively. These nurses are able to act as a conduit between clinicians and technicians.

While this situation may be satisfactory in the short term, ultimately nurses must undertake formalised education in health informatics to ensure nursing's contribution to system development and other areas of information technology implementations.

## Nursing workforce capacity

A major problem worldwide is the lack of knowledge and the capacities of the nursing workforce to use information technology to its fullest extent much less push the boundaries of the discipline. Familiarity and an understanding of the tools of nursing practice are essential and informatics is quickly becoming the most dominant of these. Nurses must be competent and confident in using these tools and able to appraise new ways of incorporating IT into their practice. In fact, Bakken, Cimino and Hripcsak, (2004) argue that informatics competences should also be integrated into employer and nursing registration requirements. This is a very large undertaking.

Building capacity in the nursing workforce is complex; on one side many nurses have no computer literacy skills and on the other there are nurses who have advanced degrees in informatics. However, the latter are the exception rather than the rule. Assumptions are made that many nurses, particularly those who have undertaken professional training in the past five years, and those who have undertaken specific systems training in individual workplaces, have some expertise (AHIC, 2004). However, figures from the Australian Institute of Health and Welfare (2005n.d.) show that the illiteracy issue will most likely continue as nurses without informatics education increased by 12 per cent from 1995 to 2001. The figures also showed that newer graduates with informatics education also decreased.

A recent comprehensive study of 2,020 nurses across a wide range of specialties and environments in the United Kingdom also places doubt on the readiness nurses to engage with IT. This study revealed that insufficient or inappropriate IT training was frequently raised by the respondents (NHS Information Authority, 2005). It ranged from none at all (60 per cent) and being expected to just 'get on with it', to being trained, but having no system or a different system in their practice area. Training was rigid and unmatched to individual learning needs. Release from the clinical area was also problematic and often 'back fill' for the ward was not provided necessitating some participants to undertake training in their own time. A participant noted: 'IT is not seen as essential when staff numbers are low' (NHS Information Authority, 2005, p. 23).

In Australia, the lack of computer knowledge of health workers is seen as impeding the realisation of the full potential of health information technology in advancing practice (Conrick, et al., 2004; General Practice Computing Group, 1999). Nursing education and training programmes at undergraduate and postgraduate levels must include NI as a core component of curricula. It is essential that beginning practitioners have base competencies in NI particularly in regard to clinical information systems. This will provide a basis for the further development of informatics knowledge and skills that must be integrated into the continued development of nursing practice.

The sheer size and disparate backgrounds of the nursing workforce makes the provision of education challenging. Undergraduates entering higher education institutions need basic computer literacy as a minimum entry standard. Governments must continue to push for a reversal in the reduction of informatics awareness in nursing and must ensure that NI competencies are incorporated in all nursing courses and offered in staff development programmes. If the nursing workforce continues to be uninformed and uneducated about informatics and its use best practice cannot be attained, and nursing, patients and their care will suffer in the long term.

## Nursing competencies

One of the key determinants for the IT skills required by nurses is the type or model of care being delivered and the areas in which they work. For instance, the requirements for those working in aged care are different from the emergency nurse, while community health workers in rural and remote Australia may not require the same skills as those working in metropolitan area.

Postgraduate qualifications in informatics provide nurses with the underlying computing concepts that they currently lack. This is not to say nurse informaticians need computer-programming skills. Rather, a solid understanding of systems development lifecycle, fundamental database concepts, network computing environments, graphical user interface design and the more technical aspects of project management would greatly enhance the individual's ability to function in rapidly changing technological environments.

In Australia, rudimentary work has begun on defining competencies although internationally nursing has been quite rigorous. A workshop conducted in 2005, demonstrated that Australian nurses might require similar competencies to the four areas surfaced in Staggers' American Delphi study (Staggers, Gassert & Curran, 2002, p. 385). The competencies are universal in nature and are presented here in a truncated version to demonstrate the major distinctions.

Beginning nurses (Level 1) have fundamental information management and computer technology skills and use existing information systems and available information to manage their practice.

Experienced nurses (Level 2) are highly skilled in using information management and computer technology skills to support their major area of practice ...

Informatics specialists (Level 3) are registered nurses prepared at least at the baccalaureate level who possess additional knowledge and skills specific to information management and computer technology … They use the tools of critical thinking, process skills, data management skills, systems development life cycle, and computer skills.

Informatics innovators (Level 4) are educationally prepared to conduct informatics research and to generate informatics theory … They understand the interdependence of systems, disciplines, and outcomes, and can finesse situations to maximize outcomes.

### The education challenge

NI remains almost invisible in undergraduate programmes, with little integration of these skills in general postgraduate nursing courses. A handful of universities offer NI at an undergraduate level, but when staff capable of teaching NI leave, they cannot be replaced and the courses are phased out. The problem in nursing education is the lack of both programmes and educational staff.

The majority of informatics programmes that now exist are at postgraduate level (Graduate Diplomas or Master) in the broader area of Health Informatics. There are comparatively few of these programmes and graduate number remains small. Some certificate programmes are offered but there are no large-scale professional training programmes in Australia at present.

One way to incorporate informatics into educational programmes for already graduated registered nurse is to integrate it into all postgraduate education. However, a sizeable percentage of clinicians have little intention of undertaking postgraduate education in informatics or any other area (Conrick, 2006b). The needs of nurses in the workforce must be met, but little incentive exists for them to gain informatics skills, as there is scant recognition of nursing informatics expertise in most employment awards. Several State Governments in Australia for instance do not recognise NI qualifications as postgraduate qualification, and no allowance is forthcoming.

### Where and why nurses must be involved in developments

Governments are interested in the effective communication of information across the continuum of care and electronic health records (EHRs) are seen as central to this. Most EHRs are adopted to create an information environment where access to information can be exploited to support care delivery, improve health outcomes, support health planning and foster further research. According to the Australian Government their Health*Connect* project will 'improve the delivery of health care and better quality of care, consumer safety and health outcomes for all Australians while enhancing the privacy and respecting the dignity of health consumer' (Commonwealth of Australia, 2000). Most of the infrastructure and infostructure being introduced into the health sector underpins a fully integrated EHR.

A range of nursing professionals will be affected by these initiatives; in particular, primary health care providers like community nurses, rural and remote nurses and nurse practitioners will be required to become regular users of national records whereas institution-based nurses will be expected to use them as part of their normal processes.

Although nurses are by far the most numerous health providers, they do not dominate health as a profession. In national records development, Australian nurses have been engaged in stakeholder committees and have had serendipitous involvement as trial managers. Although it has much to offer, nursing as a profession has not been the target of any research and development activity in the project (Conrick, et al., 2004).

These authors suggest that as key stakeholders and participants in the care delivery processes, nurses have a unique position to take lead roles in supporting the evaluation of the value, feasibility and implementation of EHRs. As a key contributor of data and most consistent user of an EHR, nurses are also well placed to be actively involved in design evaluation. This must ensure that their information needs are met and that consideration is paid to the effectiveness of nursing contributions in meeting the needs of other stakeholders. The business and data aspects of the EHR are also important and only nurses can define the business context, information flow and practices to determine what nursing information is required and only nurses can evaluate the effectiveness of this design component.

Nursing's contribution is fundamental from the technical evaluation perspective, as this must consider the ability of the infrastructure to support care delivery and fit with work practices, particularly in primary health care settings where many nurses practice. Nurses' contribution to the definition of key components of EHRs (such as the policy framework, consent models, person identification processes and access control determination) is also crucial. These components are important for both access and the appropriate flow of information. The debate on this aspect of planning will be an important change management activity. As a key stakeholder, nursing has a fundamental role in any evaluation of the effectiveness of stakeholder communications.

Nurses can offer advice on defining the building blocks of EHRs, in conjunction with other health care providers. They can ensure the applicability of these in areas such as information architecture, modelling and standards, privacy, security, unique identification, event summary definition, provider registration, central medicines repository, medication management and the development of clinical archetypes.

## 9.6 Applying nursing knowledge in a technological environment

This chapter so far has underscored the critical need for nursing to lay claim to and manage nursing information and consequently, nursing knowledge. One obvious area for the application of nursing knowledge within technological environments is the use of clinical decision support systems. Sittig (2003) describes these as comprehensive knowledge bases that are able to automatically deliver clinical guidance at the point of care within an electronic health record.

Unlike so-called expert systems that purport to replace human decision making, decision support systems are aimed at complementing the clinical skills of the clinician. They rely on sophisticated inference engines capable of applying complex sets of predetermined decision rules to well defined clinical data bases (Liaw, 1996). Such systems hold great promise in improving clinical care by reducing adverse clinical errors (Kuperman, et al., 2001, Parker, 2003). A recent review of 70 randomised controlled trials 68 per cent of clinical decision support systems demonstrated significantly improved clinical practice (Kawamoto, et al., 2005).

These authors suggest four features that lead to improved clinical practice. First, decision-support was offered automatically to the clinician as it has an inherent part of the clinical workflow. Second, rather than only assessments of clinical data, there should be a requirement for recommendations. Third, it is critical that decision support be available at the point-of-care. Finally, that decision support must be available as an inherent part of computer based clinical information systems (Kawamoto, et al., 2005).

An increasingly prevalent component of clinical information systems that use clinical decision-support are automated clinical pathways. This approach to clinical documentation requires significant nursing contribution to integrate protocol-driven evidence-based clinical documents with the underlying knowledge bases and rules engines. Clinical pathways are constructed by critically reviewing research related to a particular diagnosis or diagnostic-related group (DRG) and by analysing a significant number of patients presenting with that DRG. A series of protocols representing best practice are then built up to form the pathway. Essentially these protocols create a grid that can be used to define interventions and patient outcomes that should be achieved within predetermined time frames. Once established, they can be used for future patients with similar DRGs. If the patient deviates from the set care path in terms of required interventions or actual outcomes, a variance occurs.

Automated clinical pathways can use clinical decision support to alert clinicians when a variance occurs, allowing appropriate adjustments to the patient's care and correction in a more timely manner. Donaldson has demonstrated that using live data analysis, instead of retrospective audit, lends itself to active variance analysis and the flagging of specific indicators that predict variance during the episode of care. Adoption of his process also supports the development of most clinical pathways based on objective, empirical decisions, using the evidence of past performance. It better accommodates dynamic changes in patient conditions, enables real-time reporting and the identification of exception and/or variance for real-time quality improvements (Donaldson & Conrick, 2004).

The standardisation of concepts in clinical pathways is achieved through the integration of clinical dictionaries and clinical languages such as the Systematised Nomenclature of Medicine (SNOMED), the International Classification of Diseases (ICD-10), the North American Nursing Diagnosis Association (NANDA) or the International Classification for Nursing Practice (ICNP®). The ability of nurses to identify, classify and communicate nursing knowledge using a systematic methodology is critical to the success of these systems. However, in Australia, nursing has yet to determine a common language, and although proposals have been submitted to Government, funding for this work has not been forthcoming.

## Standardising Nursing Language

Currell, Wainwright and Urquhart (2002) recognise that nurses are key collectors, generators and users of patient/client information. However, they caution that if patient care is not consistently and accurately recorded, the possible adverse effects for the patient might be highly significant. Unless data are ordered or a classification used, the differences in nursing language can be quite marked and result in inappropriate interpretations of the patient record. This leads to the key process of nursing care being measured in different ways (Conrick, 1995).

American and European nurses have been very active in developing nursing classifications. Since 1998, the International Council of Nurses (ICN) have been developing the International Classification for Nursing Practice (ICNP® now Version one) and various national nursing organisations (including the Royal College of Nursing Australia) have supported these developments.

Several countries including Australia have decided to purchase licenses for SNOMED-CT, a terminology that claims to unambiguously represent around 350,000 concepts that are both pre- and post-coordinated. In other words, the combination of atomic concepts (e.g. 'Family History' *and* 'Breast Cancer') and multipart complex concepts expressed as a *single* phrase (e.g. 'Family history of breast cancer'). It also contains rich networks of semantic relationship links that taken together define concepts (Conrick, 2006c). Whether SNOMED-CT allows for the reliable retrieval of equivalent concepts expressed in differing ways is more contentious, and this needs to be examined further in the Australian context. Although it contains NANDA terms, the ability of SNOMED to represent nursing practice in Australia must be determined.

Scott et al., (2004) examined 70 terms and phrases of relevance to the Australian residential aged care sector and matched these to three terminologies and classifications using a five point rating scale. Inter-rater concordance for assigned rating was assessed for three author teams. After allowing for some significant biases in the study, results suggested that SNOMED CT had fair content coverage as a terminology with a 68 per cent 'hit' rate for content coverage. The Australian Classification and Terminology of Community Health (CATCH) scored a 41 per cent and as might be expected ICNP® Beta2, scored 36 per cent. This signifies an urgent need for nurses to trial languages to ensure communication across the profession and NI is essential to this process.

The standardisation of nursing language is an essential requirement for nurses across all health sectors if nursing data are to be captured in a way that it can be stored, retrieved, managed, exchanged and integrated across health care settings (Conrick, et al., 2004). It is essential if nurses are to be engaged in health informatics adoptions rather than simply swept along by it and subsumed under medical diagnoses.

However, because nursing terminologies vary across specialised areas and nursing interventions are difficult to assign terms, the standardisation of nursing language is complex and problematic (Thoroddsen, 2005). These issues prolong and impede developments of informatics tools that are capable of enabling nurses to effectively communicate across health care specialties (Simpson, 2004; Thoroddsen, 2005). Without adequate funding nursing will not be able to resolve these problems or significantly join the debate.

### Archetypes

The adoption of *open*EHR architecture to underpin Health*Connect* would reduce some of the work to be carried out in Australia and offer nursing an opportunity to describe the concepts of nursing practice for the first time. Because, fundamental to *open*EHR is the use of 'archetypes' or electronically generated documents that provide a relatively simple means for clinicians to specify the structure, content and context of clinical information without becoming involved in how programmers might represent the information within an EHR system (Conrick, et al., 2004). The *open*EHR architecture and archetypes, when implemented with appropriate software, are used to manage clinical information and knowledge in an EHR system. If *open*EHR is adopted, nursing must be responsible for the nursing knowledge contained in archetypes and should be prepared to undertake this work.

Archetypes must be underpinned by evidence based nursing practice where it exists and organisational structures, working guidelines and methodologies must also be established for the governance, naming, development, registration and distribution of nursing archetypes. This work has begun through Nursing Informatics Australia (a special interest group of the Health Informatics Society of Australia) and a web site developed to bring this work together.

## 9.7 Limitations of information technology

While much of the literature focuses on the benefits of IT in health care there are, nevertheless, some inherent limitations. Historically, information systems have been associated with significant overheads in terms of costs associated with purchase and implementation as well as time in training. Difficulties in quantifying cost savings directly related to the use of information systems in health care result in an inability to accurately determine return on investment.

In the absence of such data, health boards and executives are understandably reluctant to commit scarce financial resources to implementing these systems. In addition to the cost of acquiring the information system itself, there are enormous costs in implementing the underlying infrastructure required to drive these information systems. Many organisations do not possess the requisite network backbone to implement contemporary information systems. In most instances, the lack of appropriate clinical computing hardware and experienced informatics personnel is problematic.

If viewed from a rather limited perspective, the use of specific aspects of an information system can be seen as more time consuming than traditional methods of data acquisition. For example, it is certainly quicker for a doctor to handwrite an order for a medication or investigation than to do this using an information system. However, this short-term view ignores the potential 'downstream' timesaving and error reductions.

One frequent concern regarding the use of information systems in health care has been the potential for breaches in patient privacy and confidentiality. Some may suggest that increasing the number of clinicians who potentially have access to a record increases the risk of security breaches. The need to physically possess the traditional paper-based history largely mitigated security concerns (but this does not of course take into account the unsecured storage of paper records). Providing this information in a distributed fashion, in theory at least, increases security concerns many fold.

While it is true that patient information is more widely available using distributed technologies, it is also true that these systems possess robust authentication and authorisation processes together with stringent audit logging. Both these forms of logical security provide a level of security unattainable with traditional paper-based medical records. Every time a patient's record is accessed, a transaction is recorded and the individual clinician conducting the transaction is logged. The widespread introduction of biometric authentication will greatly enhance existing security measures.

## 9.8 The challenges for nursing

It is almost impossible for IT tools to completely align with current nursing practices; therefore, change management is essential to guide the introduction of IT into health care. Currently, the poor management of the changes that new informatics tools impose on the clinical environment hamper their uptake by nurses (Smedley, 2005). Charters (2003) advises that when introducing IT, the complexity must be reduced and steps taken to mitigate the unwanted side effects of change. The benefits must not be lost amid the adversities or challenges the change brings and during the process it is important to include both 'leaders' and 'champions' who are respected in the organisation.

Information systems must be streamlined with and not impede nurses work-flow if they are to be successfully integrated into nursing practices (Long & Long, 2005; Walsh, 2005). Unfortunately, many informatics tools have poor investments in streamlining nurses' workloads and therefore experience a poor uptake by nurses (Simpson, 2005). Nurses have a unique relationship with patients and, as discussed earlier, are the single largest collectors and users of information and data. In fact, their data input ratio is one to ten in relation to medical practitioners. Therefore, it is essential for informatics tools to offer an appealing, convenient and efficient alternative of data management to nurses (Conrick, 2003; Moss, 2005). Nurses must be involved from the beginning when planning the features of the information tools to support their workload (Conrick, 2003; Simpson, 2005).

## 9.9 Final reflection

One does not have to delve too deeply to see the array of information tools available for nurses to improve their practices and increase the quality of health care delivered to patients. The collection, storage, retrieval and communication of data in a way that promotes its transformation to information and knowledge that can be acted upon is essential to quality health care. At this time, there are two ways of looking at the slowness of governments and others to embrace nursing as central to the adoption and use of informatics in health care. First, it can be seen in terms of the paternalism of the past that has plagued the profession, making autonomy and advancement as a profession more difficult, or second, for nursing to consider the tardiness in support as providing an excellent opportunity to learn from the success and failures of other countries.

IT and informatics offers nurses the exciting prospects of describing the essence of nursing practice. In doing this they can demonstrate nursing's place in health care and nurses' valuable contributions to health outcomes. It also offers interconnectivity and communications not before seen in health care. However, the successful uptake of the tools of informatics and information management, and their subsequent benefits, are commonly impinged upon by numerous cultural, procedural, organisational, governmental, educational, technical, legal, ethical and moral factors, which must be acknowledged and addressed.

## LEARNING ACTIVITIES

1. In small groups discuss what does Nursing Informatics offer nursing?

2. List and discuss challenges created when implementing information technology into health care?

3. Discuss the politics of nursing and information technology and suggest strategies to best increase the influence and effect of nurses in this area.

## References

Anderson, J. D. (1999). Increasing the acceptance of clinical information systems. *MD Computing, 16*(1). [Retrieved 28 January 2003] http://www.mdcomputing.com/issues/

Australian Health Information Council (AHIC). (2004). *Health Workforce Health Informatics Capacity Building: National Statement 2004.* Canberra: Department of Health and Ageing.

Australian Institute of Health and Welfare (AIHW). (n.d.). *Data Collection Systems.* [Retrieved 12 April 2005] httpa//:ww4v.aihw.gov.au/publicationsihwi/

Bakken, S., Cimino, J. & Hripcsak, G. (2004). Promoting patient safety and enabling evidence-based practice through informatics. *Medical Care, 42*(2), 49–56.

Ball, M. (2001). Nursing informatics in USA: New opportunities, new responsibilities. *British Journal of Healthcare Computing & Information Management, 18*(6), 21–23.

Ball, M., Gulinson, G., Hannah, K., Hersher, B. & Smith, C. (2000). Bedside to boardroom: New challenges for nursing informatics leaders. In Saba, V., Carr, R., Sermus, W., & Rocha, P. (eds), *One Step Beyond: The Evolution of Technology and Nursing.* Auckland: Adis International, pp. 237–242.

Borthwick, C. & Galbally, R. (2001). Nursing leadership and health sector reform. *Nursing Inquiry, 8*(2), 75–81.

Boston Consulting Group. (2004). *National Health Information Management and Information and Communications Technology Strategy.* Australian Health Information Council. Canberra.

Charters, K. (2003). Nursing informatics, outcomes, and quality improvement. *Clinical Issues: Advanced Practice in Acute and Critical Care, 14*(3), 282–294.

CHIK Services. (2004). *Australian eHealth Market: Acute Care 2003–2005.* Gosford, CHIK Services Pty Ltd.

Chu, S. (2001). Computerised clinical pathway management systems and the implications. *Collegian, 8*(2), 19–24.

Commonwealth of Australia. (2000). *National Electronic Records Taskforce.* Canberra: Department of Health and Ageing.

Conrick, M. (1995). *Issues in Informatics: Nursing within Health* (Vol. 1). Brisbane: Centre for Research Griffith University.

Conrick, M. (2003). Nursing and the electronic health record. Presentation at the *Nursing in a Technological World Conference,* Hilton Hotel, Brisbane: July 1–4.

Conrick, M. (2005). Nursing Informatics. In Funnell, R., Koutoukidis, G. & Lawrence, K. (eds), *Tabbner's Nursing Care* (4th edn.). Melbourne: Elsivier Churchill Livingstone.

Conrick, M. (2006a). Informatics Professional Roles and Governance. In M. Conrick (ed.), *Health Informatics: Transforming Healthcare with Technology.* Melbourne: Thompson Publishing, pp. 290–300.

Conrick, M. (2006b). Workforce capacity building. In M. Conrick (ed.), *Health informatics: Transforming healthcare with technology.* Melbourne: Thompson Publishing, pp. 300–310.

Conrick, M., Hovenga, E., Cook, R., Laracuente, T. & Morgan, T. (2004). *A Framework for Nursing Informatics in Australia: A Strategic Paper.* Melbourne: Department of Health and Ageing.

Conrick, M., Walker, S., Scott, P. & Frean, I. (2006c). Health Information Interchange. In M. Conrick (ed.), *Health Informatics: Transforming Healthcare with Technology.* Melbourne: Thompson Publishing, pp. 20–39.

Cox, M. (2003). What are the implications of Information Technology on nursing and how might it impact the nursing shortage? Proceedings of the *HIC2003 & RACGP 12CC Conference,* Sydney. 10–12 August.

Currell, R., Wainwright, P. & Urquhart, C. (2002). *Nursing Record Systems: Effects on Nursing Practice and Healthcare Outcomes.* Oxford: The Cochrane Library Update Software.

Donaldson, P., & Conrick, M. (2004). *The Effectiveness Of Using A Patient Dependency System To Develop And Audit Clinical Pathways.* Paper presented at the HIC2004, Brisbane.

Economist looks at the barriers to Health IT. (2005). (05 May). *Economist,* p. 45.

Englebardt, S. & Nelson, R. (2002). *Healthcare Informatics: An Interdisciplinary Approach.* Sydney: Mosby Inc.

General Practice Computing Group. (1999). *Survey of Information Technology Activities in the Australian Divisions of General Practice.* Barton: Australian Medical Association.

Hall, L. M., Doran, D. & Pink, G. H. (2004). Nurse staffing models, nursing hours, and patient safety outcomes. *Journal of Nursing Administration, 34*(1), 41–45.

Herlihy, R. & Allen, M. (2005). Building the compelling case to invest in nursing documentation. Proceedings *National Health Informatics Conference.* Melbourne. 31 July–2 August.

Hersher, B. (2000). New roles for nurses in healthcare information systems. In Ball, M. J., Hannah, K. J., Newbold, S. K., & Douglas, J. V. (eds), *Nursing Informatics: Where Caring and Technology Meet* (3rd edn.). New York: Springer-Verlag, pp. 264–283.

HISA. (1998). *Definition of Health Informatics.* [Retrieved 5 October 2004] http://hisa.org.au

Huges, S. J. (2000). Point of care information systems: State of the art. In Ball, M. J., Hannah, K. J., Newbold, S. K. & Douglas, J. V. (eds), *Computers in Healthcare Nursing Informatics: Where Caring and Technology Meet* (2nd edn.). New York: Springer-Verlag, pp. 242–252.

IMIA-NI. (1998). *Definition*. [Retrieved February 4, 2003] http://www.imia.org/

International Medical Informatics Association. (2000). *Recommendations of the International Medical Informatics Association (IMIA) on Education in Health and Medical Informatics.* [Retrieved 10 April 2005] http://www.imia.org/

Kawamoto, K., Houlihan, C. A., Balas, E. A. & Lobach, D. F. (2005). Improving clinical practice using clinical decision support systems: a systematic review of trials to identify features to success. *British Medical Journal, 330,* 76.

Kirkley, D. & Stein, M. (2004). Nurses and clinical technology: Sources of resistance and strategies for acceptance. *Nursing Economics, 22*(4), 216–223.

Kuperman, G. J., Teich, J. M., Gandhi, T. K. & Bates, D. W. (2001). Patient safety and computerised medication ordering at Brigham and Women's Hospital. *Joint Commission Journal on Quality Improvement, 27*(10), 509–521.

Liaw, T. (1996). Decision Support in Clinical Practice. In Hovenga, E., Kidd, M. & Cesnik, B. (eds). *Health Informatics: An Overview*. South Melbourne: Churchill Livingstone, pp. 161–172.

Lipp, A. & Williams, C. (2002). The implementation of a computerised clinical information system: with a view to care. *Journal of Neonatal Nursing, 8*(5), 162–165.

Long, L. & Long, N. (2005). *Computers* (12th edn.). Sydney: Prentice Hall.

McCartney, P. R. (2004). Leadership in nursing informatics. *Journal of Obstetric, Gynecologic, and Neonatal Nursing, 33*(3), 371–380.

McKeown, P. G. (2001). *Information Technology and the Networked Economy*. Fort Worth, Texas: Harcourt College Publishers.

Moss, J. (2005). Technological system solutions to clinical communication error. *Journal of Nursing Administration, 35*(2), 51–53.

National Health Service. (2003). *Health Informatics Competency Profiles for the National Health Service*. [Retrieved 22 February 2005] http://www.nelh.nhs.uk/

Parker, P. (2003). Computerised order entry goes beyond safety net. *Nursing Management, 34*(2), 45–46.

PricewaterhouseCoopers LLP. (2005). *Reactive to Adaptive: Transforming Hospitals with Digital Technology*. Delaware: PricewaterhouseCoopers.

Proctor, P. M. (2000). Apocalypse-shortly. In Saba, V., Carr, R., Sermus, W., & Rocha, P. (eds), *One Step beyond: The Evolution of Technology and Nursing.* Auckland: Adis International, pp. 39–44

Protti, D. J. (2005). *The Use of Computers in Healthcare can Reduce Errors, Improve Patient Safety and Enhance the Quality of Service-There is Evidence*. National Programme for IT in the NHS. [Retrieved 25 June 2005] http://www.connectingforhealth.nhs.uk/

Reinecke, I. (2005, May). Australia's e-Health Agenda: What it means for older Australians. Presentation at the *National Aged Care Informatics Conference*, Hobart, Tasmania.

Saba, V. (2001). Nursing informatics: Yesterday, today and tomorrow. *International Nursing Review, 48*(3), 177–187.

Scott, P., Jones, L., Saad, P., Conrick, M., Foster, J. & Campbell, M. (2004). *Matching Residential Aged Care Terms to SNOMED CT, ICNP2Beta, and CATCH.* Presentation at the *ACCIC04 Conference*, Brisbane.

Silver, D. (2002). Doing away with paper: Part 1 – advice for setting up fully computerised medical records. *Australian Family Physician, 31*(6), 521–526, 551, 553 *passim.*

Sim, I., Sanders, G. & McDonald, K. (2002). Evidence-based practice for mere mortals. *Journal of General Internal Medicine, 17,* 302–308.

Simpson, R. (2004). The softer side of technology: How IT helps nursing care. *Nursing Administration Quarterly, 28*(4), 302–305.

Simpson, R. (2005). Patient and nurse safety: How information technology makes a difference. *Nursing Administration Quarterly, 29*(1), 97–101.

Sittig, D. F (2003). An Overview of efforts to bring clinical knowledge to the point of care. Proceedings *Second National Health Informatics and Management Conference.* Auckland New Zealand. 6–8 August.

Smedley, A. (2005). The importance of informatics competencies in nursing: An Australian perspective. *CIN: Computers, Informatics, Nursing, 23*(2), 106–110.

Staggers, N., Gassert, C. & Curran, C. (2002). A Delphi study to determine informatics competencies for nurses at four levels of practice. *Nursing Research, 51*(6), 383–390.

Thoroddsen, A. (2005). Applicability of the nursing interventions classification to describe nursing. *Scandinavian Journal Caring Science,* 19, 128–139.

Tsuru, S. & Yasuaki, F. (2000). Economic value of nursing information: Pecuniary value of the nursing summary. In Saba, V., Carr, R., Sermus, W., & Rocha, P. (eds), *One Step Beyond: The Evolution of Technology and Nursing.* Auckland: Adis International, pp. 461–467.

Unruh, L.Y. & Byers, J. F. (2002). Hospital downsizing: International experiences and perspectives. *Nursing and Health Policy Review, 1*(2), 117–151.

Van de Velde, R. & Degoulet, P. (2003). *Clinical Information Systems: A Component Based Approach.* New York: Springer-Verlag.

Walsh, S. (2005). Turn it on you expect it to work. *Health Matters, 10*(4), 7.

## RECOMMENDED READING

Coiera, E. (2003). *Guide to Health Informatics* (2nd edn.). London: Arnold.

Conrick, M. (2006). *Health Informatics: Transforming Healthcare with Technology.* Melbourne: Thompson Publishing.

Darbyshire, P. (2000). The practice politics of computerised information systems: A focus group study. *Nurse Researcher, 8*(2), 4–17.

Hebda, T., Czar, P. & Mascara, C. (2005). *Handbook of Informatics for Nurses and Health Care Professionals* (3rd edn.). Upper Saddle River, NJ: Pearson Prentice Hall.

Romano, C.A. (1990). Innovation: The promise and the perils for nursing and information technology. *Computers in Nursing, 8*(3), 99–104.

# Technological Change and Nursing: A Labour Process Theory Approach to the Shaping of Nursing Work

10

---

## Carol Windsor

---

From a reading of this chapter, you will be able to:

- Discuss labour process theory
- Consider how the concept of technology is addressed in nursing literature
- Identify changes in the structure of nursing work
- Understand arguments relating to the shaping of nursing work
- Address the role of the state in the regulation of nursing work

---

- capitalism
- de-skilling
- division of labour
- multi-skilling
- nursing

- productivity

- specialisation

- technology

## 10.1 Nursing and the labour process

A point of departure in this chapter is that technologies and technological change in nursing cannot be treated separately from an understanding of nursing work as socially defined, shaped and organised. Accounts of nursing work typically focus on work *within* nursing where studies focus on, for example, the occupational socialisation of nurses (Melia, 1987); relations with doctors, patients and others (Savage, 1995); and specific skills and practices (Latimer, 1997). Or they specify a political identity for nursing work such as professional labour (Walby & Soothill, 1994), emotional or caring labour (Davies, 1995a) and gendered labour (Davies, 1995b). Few studies of nursing work have treated it as *work* that is organised in relation to the wider structural impulses that govern the production and reproduction of the intellectual and material practices of labour. Those that have (Allen, 2001; Strauss, et al., 1997) have tended to set out empirical studies of nursing in specific organisational settings.

This chapter treats nursing work as *work* and examines the effects of broader institutional and organisational change on nursing practice. It addresses an approach derived from political economy (Braverman, 1974) that seeks to understand nursing work in the context of intensively organised and regulated production of material practice. To frame this discussion of nursing work and its new technologies of practice we address contemporary approaches to technological development in nursing and the limitations of such works in explaining the role of technology in nursing and specifically in the changing division of nursing labour and the principle drivers of such change.

It is argued that introducing Braverman's labour process theory makes it possible to understand nursing in a wider context, not simply as gendered labour, but as *work* defined by capitalist production. Having established the relevance of this approach, we then explore ways in which the state, not as an exogenous or neutral body but as essentially capitalist, mediates changes to work organisation in relation to interventions that increasingly act to regulate and structure nursing work.

From this perspective, we point to the ways that reviews on nursing work and nursing policies are framed and organised to socially and politically reshape nursing work. Technologies are central to this, since they define, mobilise and act to integrate new forms of health care delivery and ways of working in the interests of productivity demands. An appeal to technological and knowledge development is crucial to the organisation of nursing work and we see how this discourse acts as a regulatory strategy imposed upon nurses and nursing.

## 10.2 Health technologies and divisions of labour: Routinisation and specialisation

The popular view is that the recent appearance of more technologically complex health care has increased the demand for nurses to be functionally flexible and to demonstrate higher levels of competencies. It appears, therefore, that it has become technically necessary for the nursing labour force to upgrade skills in response to technological change (Simpson, 2005) to embrace, not resist, technological change (Kirkley & Stein, 2004; Timmons, 2003) to optimise the use of technology to improve productivity; and to counter labour shortages (Bower & McCullough, 2004; Meadows, 2002; Simpson, 2004; Slocumb, 2005) and to be 'innately' adaptable to technological developments (DEST, 2002).

The assumption central to such views is that nursing work is being transformed in fundamental ways through the impact of new technologies on work structures. New technologies have created new demands and challenges in nursing, and these, in turn, require the adjustment of nurses to productive activity. The education and skills of nurses must be upgraded and roles redesigned in a constant drive to optimise the possibilities of technological innovation.

The link between technological change and 'up-skilling' in nursing is a variant of a broader argument that sees the more recent technological developments linked to the appearance of the 'knowledge worker' within a 'new information economy'. A feature of this argument is that we are witnessing a shift towards a new paradigm of work (an information society) that calls for a more flexible and better educated workforce. Writers such as Piore and Sabel (1984), and more recently Castells (1996) and Giddens (2000), suggest that the autonomy required by new technologies is producing a 'learning economy' and multi-skilled occupations and, within these, workers who enjoy unprecedented control over their work. The implication is that work and knowledge need to be restructured to meet the requirements of a 'new economy'.

Yet such works pose a universality of the technological trend that is inadequate in explaining the ways in which the nature of nursing work is being transformed. Both the definitions of nursing tasks and their division between workers are shaped, in part, by knowledge and technologies. For example, new technologies may have empowered some sectors within nursing where greater specialisation has seen higher remuneration of technical skills (see the Buchan and Calman 2004 OECD survey of various advance practice nursing roles). But there is no universality to this trend and nor in the way that nursing work is organised (or is being reorganised). Indeed, what we observe in nursing is a move towards greater occupational diversification. Nursing labour is being increasingly casualised (AIHW, 2002), the roles of assistant nurses/carers are expanding (Daykin & Clarke, 2000) and more specialised roles such as the nurse practitioner (or advanced practitioner) (Buchan & Calman, 2004) and the 'telenurse' (Greenburg, 2000) are developing. It is the emergence of new categories of workers in nursing and the increasing variability in the nature of nursing work that the determinist arguments of proponents of the technologically driven 'knowledge worker' cannot account for (nor explain).

We need, therefore, to shift the discussion to the much neglected issue of the division of nursing labour and the ways in which nursing work is constantly revolutionised in response and in the first instance, not to technology, but to the competitive relations of capitalism. This means locating technological change and its impact on the organisation of nursing work within a context of a broader political economy. We understand that in the process of the transformation of capitalist productive forces, technological development becomes the instrument whereby jobs, division of labour and technical skills requisites are continually altered.

The starting point of analysis is the concrete reality of capitalism and the labour process. Here we turn to Braverman's (1974) *Labour and Monopoly Capital*, a seminal work that focused attention on the workplace and the political nature of technological change. Braverman argued that the structural requirements of twentieth-century capitalism had brought about the degregation of work through the processes of deskilling. Deskilling refers to the fragmentation of work where the skill content required by any one worker is reduced and the result is cheaper labour and the ultimate subordination of workers to the control of management. As Braverman (1974, p. 81) argues, this occurs where the labour process is

> separated into elements some of which are simpler than others and each of which is simpler than the whole. Translated into market terms this means that the labour power capable of performing the process may be purchased more cheaply as dissociated elements than as a capacity integrated in a single worker.

Braverman refers to this process as the separation of the conception and execution of work where managers take over the conception of work and non-managers execute detailed tasks as directed. The means by which the fragmentation of work is achieved is through technological innovation. Technological advance leads to greater control over the work process through specialisation of work and removal of decision making from the worker. Technology is understood, in this sense, not as a neutral entity, but as fundamentally capitalist. In other words, it is the requirements and interests of capitalist production that compel technological development and its application.

There has been much critique and refinement of Braverman's thesis (Carter, 1997; Thompson, 1990; Thomson & Smith, 2001) and most notably because of the emphasis on de-skilling, loss of autonomy and lessening job control. Yet, Braverman addressed this issue in arguing that the subordination of workers in the production process 'is an ideal realized by capital only within definite limits, and unevenly among industries' (1974, p. 172). Furthermore, 'its very application brings into being new crafts and skills and technical specialties which are at first the province of labour rather than management' (1974, p. 172). In Braverman's analysis, technological innovation requires, if only temporarily, the development of new skills and competencies (Spencer, 2000). Indeed and as noted above, we see that changes in nursing work content are variable in lowering the requisite skills of some who carry out nursing work and upgrading the skills of others. Hence, conditions of relative autonomy and tight control co-exist in nursing settings (Bolton, 2004) and there is no claim therefore to a uniform tendency towards deskilling. It is also argued that the emphasis on managerialism in Braverman's work shifts the analysis away from the broader economic and institutional structures that characterise capitalism (Jaros, 2001). Yet, the contention here is that Braverman's concern with the general tendency towards the degradation of work as a (non-linear) feature of advanced capitalism still holds relevance for a discussion of the nursing labour force.

## 10.3 From professionalisation to flexibility

The real problem with the concepts of the 'knowledge worker' and 'information society' is that they are patently at odds with the reality of the nursing workplace. The recent evolution of the division of nursing labour is vividly illustrated by contrasting the current situation with that of the 1970s and 1980s. The earlier period was significant because it appeared that the long struggle in nursing for the higher order status of a professional occupation might finally be successful through investment in education and new forms of work activity. Work was to be transformed from a largely technical role where nurses carried out certain activities according to level of training, into a form of care where the registered nurse assumed responsibility for the psychological and social as well as the physical aspects of illness. This meant that nursing work was no longer to be considered as a series of fragmented tasks allocated on the basis of hierarchy (Short, Sharman & Speedy, 1998). Instead nursing work had to be recognised as care for the whole 'patient' and the sole responsibility of the nurse. Thus the promise of the professionalisation agenda was to assert the autonomy of nurses and to ensure jurisdiction over the occupational area by redefining nursing work. The dominant discourse of this agenda was centred on individualised (or 'holistic') care and the nurse – patient therapeutic relationship.

Yet, decades later this promise remains largely unrealised. Nursing work has significantly restructured but the result is a greater degree of polarisation in skill levels, a trajectory that bears little resemblance to the professionalisation project. This process, or a differentiation in work activity, is commonly referred to as 'changing skill mix' and involves (in contrast to the Piore and Sabel thesis) the redistribution of functions of nursing work across a range of staff with varying qualifications. Highly specialised and low-skilled routinised work functions increasingly co-exist in nursing but with a disproportionate rate of growth in the latter form of work. For example, over the period 1996 to 2001 in Australia, the registered nurse/midwife sector grew by 7.3 per cent and the nursing assistant/ personal carer sector by 18.8 per cent (Productivity Commission, 2005). Thus, despite the emphasis on the 'new learning economy', we see the emergence of increasing numbers of low skilled nursing jobs. This is, as Thompson and Smith (2001) note, characteristic of all industries where the fastest growing jobs are located at the bottom of the occupational ladder and where tasks are frequently repetitive, standardised and highly controlled. Indeed, Flanagan (1998) refers to this trend and as it appears in nursing, as a necessary imperative of 'postmodern' world of flexible work. In this world, Flanagan (1998) argues, nursing requires relatively small numbers of highly skilled and knowledgeable workers, a 'technical or knowledge elite'.

We see, therefore, a shift in professional nursing discourse where care of the patient is no longer considered the reserved territory of nurses and holistic care is replaced by the concepts of flexibility, multi-skilling and teamwork. As Buchan and Dal Poz (2002) point out, a focus in the nursing literature on care as the exclusive role of registered nurses, while prominent (and mainly in the US) up until the late-1980s, has virtually disappeared. Focus has since shifted markedly to various examinations of the substitution of registered nurses by less qualified or unqualified workers (Adams, et al., 2000; Daykin & Clarke, 2000; Rheaume, 2003), the appearance of new specialist roles (Buchan & Calman, 2004) and the casualisation of the nursing workforce (Creegan, Duffield & Forrester, 2003; De Rutyer, 2004; Richardson & Allen, 2001).

A distinctive feature of this shift is the role of the state in positioning technological development as the basis for change in the occupational composition of nursing. The 'state' is a largely un-theorised concept in nursing literature. Yet, state intervention has been vital throughout the history of nursing in regulating work, education and wages. In other words and although the division of nursing labour has certainly been constructed in part by technique and knowledge, this is not to say that it has evolved in an unmediated fashion. Stimulated by capitalism's relentless pursuit of productivity gains, the state facilitates policies that ensure the more efficient use of labour. Thus, in invoking the labour process theory, we understand the state, not as an autonomous entity, but as a capitalist state that functions as 'guarantor of the conditions (and) social relations, of capitalism' (Braverman, 1974, p. 284). In nursing and as argued above, the most recent manifestation of the productivity-driven agenda has been the intensified technical division of nursing labour. As we see below, both the capitalist state and technological and knowledge development have been crucial factors in the imposition of new regulatory working conditions upon nurses and nursing.

## 10.4 The State and the Productivity Agenda

The pursuit of micro-economic reform, as part of a broader productivity and competition agenda, has been a persuasive force in health care sectors over recent decades (Adams, et al., 2000; Bolton, 2004; Productivity Commission, 2005). Even though productivity in the service sector cannot be adequately measured (Bryan & Rafferty, 1999), it is assumed that productivity gains are ensured if the cost of provision of services is lowered. This standard economic presumption has seen a concerted drive for greater efficiencies in health care through workplace flexibility, resulting in an emphasis on reducing the cost of labour (for example, by deskilling and increased casualisation) for the purposes of managing budgets. The shift is reflected in key policy documents that give support to multi-skilling and flexibility and therefore a more malleable nursing workforce.

In the United Kingdom, *Making a Difference*, a government policy statement on the future of nursing and midwifery, proposed a 'new' and flexible nursing model, a central feature of which is the introduction of the vocational roles of nursing and midwife cadets (DoH, 1999). An Australian Government initiative which culminated in the 2002 *Australian National Review of Nursing Education* argues the need for a more 'appropriate' and sustainable skill mix in the delivery of nursing care where 'the different skills of different groups can be best organised to ensure optimum outcomes for patients/clients' (DEST, 2002, p. 13). In terms reminiscent of Braverman, the Review notes that that greater skill mix will ensure the more effective use of the 'higher order' skills of professional nurses.

The major justification for the reforms outlined in both documents is the perceived need for a 'richer' skill mix of nursing workers as a response to both the current nursing labour shortage and a rapid growth in technology and knowledge. Yet, two points are noted about the agenda underlying these policy statements.

First, a shortage of nursing labour is not a new phenomenon but has been a historical feature of nursing. The theme of nursing shortages is evident throughout the twentieth century. For example, the American Nurses Association in 1920 (King, 1989), the Trained Nurses' Guild in Australia in 1922 (Trembath & Hellier, 1987), the NSW Kelly Report of 1943 and the US 1948 *Report for National Nursing Council* (Brown, 1948) all pointed to 'current' difficulties in attracting and retaining nursing staff. In the United Kingdom, the Lancet (1932), Wood (1947) and Briggs (1972) reports were all similarly focused on issues related to nursing shortages. The point to be made here is that the current labour shortage in nursing does not explain the relatively recent focus on multi-skilling, flexibility and productivity; first, because of the historical persistence of shortages in nursing and second because efficiency, flexibility and job redesign policies are being adopted across industries. As Braverman (1974, p. 82) argues, it is in the 'the mythology of capitalism' that the fragmentation of work (or production) is presented as a necessary response to skill shortages where the more specialist skills need to be used efficiently and for the overall social good.

A second point is that recent policies, as noted above, invoked in the name of technological development treat technology as an autonomous and exogenous force and neglect the nature of change within capitalist economies and the workplace. Here technology is treated as a phenomenon that signals a 'new era' or a break with the past and nurses, in this sense, become the passive objects of technical change. Nursing work is changed by technology and nurses must adapt to and accommodate such change. But this assumes a direct causal relationship between the appearance of new technologies and the restructuring of nursing work. Again, we return to policy documents of two or three decades past and we see that 'rapid advances in technology' appears as a recurring factor in arguments for the reform of nursing education and the 'upskilling' of nursing work (see for example in relation to Australia; RANF, 1971, College of Nursing, 1974, Queensland Board of Advanced Education, 1976, ALP, 1980). A shared premise of such documents is that the 'technological and scientific revolutions' (RANF, 1971) that had driven rapid change in health care provision demanded of nurses higher intellectual and practical skills. Importantly, part of this 'upskilling' agenda was the drive for the recognition of a single level practitioner, the registered nurse. As the International Nursing Council recommended in 1986: 'until the goal of an all-registered nurse staff is achieved, a second category of nursing personnel be retained but that the numbers be progressively scaled down concomitantly with the measures to increase the number of registered nurses' (RANF Queensland Branch Council Minutes, January, 1988).

This brings to our attention a disjuncture that challenges the conceptual coherence of much nursing literature on technology and nursing. On the one hand, there is a remarkable and historical continuity in the appeal to technological development as the basis for restructuring nursing. On the other hand, there is as just a remarkable discontinuity in the manner that nursing work is addressed. If we take the policy documents noted above as a whole, it is not the appearance of a technological and knowledge revolution that signals (at any historical point) a 'new era' or some significant shift in nursing. Rather, the point of departure in both the earlier and current periods is the construction of nursing work. If there has been a shift, it is from what Flanagan (1998, pp. 131–132) refers to as the ideal of the 'purist professionalisers, who would wish for an all qualified nursing workforce', to a definition of the nursing workforce (and by implication of nurse and nursing work) that now encompasses all the 'different groups who form the team of people doing nursing or care work' (DEST, 2002, p. 13).

We see, therefore, that changes in the structure of nursing work are not to be understood as simply either a response to a nursing labour 'crisis' or to some new and profound technological transformation. A preoccupation with these issues suggests a periodisation of the history of nursing that obscures the evolutionary relationship between technical progress, division of labour and capitalist production. In returning to Braverman's labour process theory, we see technical progress as a historical tendency that ensures the division of labour and if applied to nursing, recent trends as an acceleration of this process. Technologies allow for the modification and improvement of labour productivity through both increased specialisation and the sub-division of work.

## 10.5 Final reflection

The intent of this chapter is not merely to engage in a critique of the proponents of the 'new technological and knowledge economy' but to bring a focus to the logic of capitalism production and the ways in which technical progress or technological development allows and induces subdivision, specialisation and differentiation of nursing work. A key proposition is that productivity, by the means of technical progress and division of labour, is intrinsic to the determining motive of capitalism, namely the pursuit of profit. In this sense, new technologies allow the segmentation of nursing work and this occurs because it supports the specific requirements of capitalism. As Braverman (1974, p. 82) argues, 'The capitalist mode of production systematically destroys all-round skills where they exist, and brings into being skills and occupations that correspond to its needs'.

Thus, the objective has been to challenge the view that a 'major technological paradigm' shift has taken place resulting in a trend towards higher skills for all nurses and a qualitative change in the nature of nursing work. There are on-going changes in the patterns of nursing work organisation but there is considerable evidence that this is resulting in an intensified division of nursing labour and thus a far from universal increase in the levels of skill and autonomy of nurses. The general argument has been, therefore, that while technological and knowledge development clearly has an impact on nursing work, it does not of itself explain an increasing divergence in job content and subsequently earnings and opportunities in nursing.

It has further been argued that the demands for increased productivity and the presumption of flexibility are not the decisions of nurses but are imposed upon nursing. Indeed, the resultant changing division of labour has meant that the burdens of greater flexibility (casualisation) and multi-skilling (deskilling) fall squarely on nursing workers. The problem central to the claim of a 'technological' or 'knowledge' revolution is, therefore, that it presents the transformation of nursing work as inevitable and 'natural' and in so doing depoliticises the costs and gains of such change. The cost of such change in nursing is a deskilling of nurses who work at the frontline of nursing care provision. An arguable gain, and as has been pointed out, is the appearance of new specialisations in nursing such as the various advanced practice roles. Yet, the very co-existence of conditions of 'upskilling' and 'deskilling' in nursing suggests that the competitive and productivity agenda (the appeal to a sustainable workforce) and the regulatory structures it imposes prevails. The implication here is that an effective politicisation (or re-politicisation) of nursing requires not only an analysis of the current trends in the technical division of nursing labour but also a historical account of the ways in which technologies, division of labour and the state have shaped nursing work.

### LEARNING ACTIVITIES

1. Structure a debate around the issue of nursing and politics. A critical question is whether nurses and nursing can be an influential political force and why/why not?

2. In a group discuss the issue of the nursing division of labour and consider how technology has/has not contributed to the structure of nursing work.

3. In a group, discuss the merits or otherwise of the concept of a 'nursing technical elite'.

# References

Adams, A., Lugsden, E., Chase, J., Arber, S. & Bond, S. (2000). Skill-Mix changes and work intensification in nursing. *Work, Employment and Society.* 14(3), 541–555.

Australian Institute of Health and Welfare (AIHW). (2002). *Nursing Labour Force.* Australian Government Printing Services, Canberra.

Allen, D. (2001). *The Changing Shape of Nursing Practice: The Role of Nurses in the Hospital Division of Labour.* London: Routledge.

Australian Labor Party (ALP). (1980). *A New Deal for Nurses. Needs in Education Series.* Prepared by John Button and Neal Blewett. RANF Queensland Branch.

Bolton, S. C. (2004). A Simple matter of control? NHS Hospital nurses and new management. *Journal of Management Studies,* 41(2), 317–333.

Bower, F. L. & McCullogh, C. (2004). Nurse shortage or nursing shortage: Have we missed the real problem? *Nursing Economics,* 22(4), 200–203.

Braverman, H. (1974). *Labor and Monopoly Capital: The Degradation of Work in the Twentieth Century.* London: Monthly Review Press.

Briggs, A. (1972). Report of the committee of nursing. HMSO, London.

Brown, E. L. (1948). *Nursing for the Future A Report Prepared for the National Nursing Council.* Russell Sage Foundation, New York.

Bryan, D. & Rafferty, M. (1999). *The Global Economy in Australia.* Australia: Allen and Unwin.

Buchan, J. & Calman, L. (2004). *Skill-Mix and Policy Change in the Health Workforce: Nurses in Advanced Roles.* Working Paper No. 17, OECD, Paris.

Buchan, J. & Dal Poz, M. R. (2002). Skill mix in the health care workforce: Reviewing the evidence. *Bulletin of the World Health Organisation,* 80(7), 575–580.

Carter, B. (1997). Restructuring state employment. *Capital and Class. Autumn 63,* 65–84.

Castells, M. (1996). *The Rise of the Network Society.* Oxford: Blackwell.

College Of Nursing (1974). *A Report on Possible Redevelopments in Nurse Education for Queensland.* College of Nursing, Australia.

Creegan, R., Duffield, C. & Forrester, K. (2003). Casualisation of the nursing workforce in Australia: Driving forces and implications. *Australian Health Review,* 26(1), 201–208.

Davies C. (1995a). Competence versus care? Gender and caring work revisited. *Acta Sociologica* 38, 17–32.

Davies C. (1995b). *Gender and the Professional Predicament in Nursing.* Buckingham: Open University Press.

Daykin N. & Clarke B. (2000). 'They'll still get the bodily care'. Discourses of care and relationships between nurses and healthcare assistants in the NHS. *Sociology of Health and Illness,* 22, 349–363.

Department of Education, Science and Training (DEST). (2002). *National Review of Nursing Education 2002: Our Duty of Care.* Canberra, Australia.

Department of Health (DoH). (1999). *Making a Difference: Strengthening the Nursing, Midwifery and Health Visiting Contribution to Health and Health Care.* HMSO, London.

De Rutyer, A. (2004). Casual work in nursing and other clinical professions: Evidence from Australia. *Journal of Nursing Management,* 12, 62–68.

Flanagan, J. (1998). Achieving partnership: The contribution of nursing education to the production of a flexible workforce. *Journal of Nursing Management,* 6, 129–136.

Giddens, A. (2000). *The Third Way and its Critics.* Cambridge: Polity Press.

Greenberg, M. E. (2000). The domain of telenursing: Issues and prospects. *Nursing Economics,* 18(4), 220–224.

Jaros, S. (2001). Labour process theory: A commentary on the debate. *International Studies of Management and Organisation,* 30(4), 25–39.

King, M. G. (1989). Nursing shortage, circa 1915. *Image: Journal of Nursing Scholarship, 21*(3), 124–127.

Kirkley, D. & Stein, M. (2004). Nurses and clinical technology: Sources of resistance and strategies for acceptance. *Nursing Economics, 22*(4), 216–222.

Lancet Commission of Nursing. (1932). *Inquiry into the Reasons for the Shortage of Nursing.* London: Lancet Ltd.

Latimer, J. (1997). Giving patients a future: The constituting of classes in an acute medical unit. *Sociology of Health and Illness, 19,* 160–185.

Meadows, G. (2002). The nursing shortage: Can information technology help? *Nursing Economics, 20*(1), 46–48.

Melia, K. (1987). *Learning and Working: The Occupational Socialization of Nurses.* London: Tavistock Publications Ltd.

Piore, M. & Sabel, C. (1984). *The Second Industrial Divide: Possibilities for Prosperity.* New York: Basic Books.

Productivity Commission. (2005). *Australia's Health Workforce.* Position Paper, Canberra.

Queensland Board of Advanced Education. (1976). *Report of Committee to Advise on Desirable Developments in Nursing Education.* Queensland. (The Livingstone Report).

RANF. (1971). *Report of the Committee of Inquiry into Nursing.* Queensland Branch, Brisbane. (The Saint Report).

RANF. (1988). *Educational and Professional Activities Committee* Report of the Meeting 18 January, Queensland.

Rheaume, A. (2003). The changing division of labour between nurses and nursing assistants in New Brunswick. *Journal of Advanced Nursing, 41*(5), 435–443.

Richardson, S. & Allen, J. (2001). Casualisation of the nursing workforce: A New Zealand perspective on an international phenomenon. *International Journal of Nursing Practice, 7,* 104–108.

Savage, J. (1995). *Nursing Intimacy: An Ethnographic Approach to Nurse–Patient Interaction.* Harrow: Scutari Projects Ltd.

Short, S., Sharman, E. & Speedy, S. (1998). *Sociology for Nurses.* South Yarra, Victoria: MacMillan.

Simpson, R. L. (2005). Practice to evidence to practice: Closing the loop with IT. *Nursing Management, 9,* 12–17.

Simpson, R. L. (2004). Recuit, retain, assess technology's role in diversity. *Nursing Administration Quarterly, 28*(3), 217–220.

Slocumb, E. M. (2005). Information technology: Supporting the practice of nurses. *The Florida Nurse, 3,* 24.

Spencer, D. A. (2000). Braverman and the contribution of labour process analysis to the critique of capitalist production – twenty-five years on. *Work, Employment and Society, 14*(2), 223–243.

Strauss, A., Fagerhough, S., Suczek, B. & Wiener, C. (1997). *Social Organization of Medical Work.* London: Transaction.

Thompson, P. (1990). Crawling from the Wreckage: The labour process and the politics of production. In D. Knights & H. Willmott (eds), *Labour Process Theory.* London: Macmillan, pp. 95–124.

Thompson, P. & Smith, C. (2001). Follow the Redbrick Road. *International Studies of Management and Organisation, 30*(4), 40–67.

Timmons, S. (2003). Nurses resisting information technology. *Nursing Inquiry, 10*(4), 257–269.

Tembath, R. & Hellier, D. (1987). *All Care and Responsibility A History of Nursing in Victoria 1850–1934.* The Florence Nightingale Committee, Australia, Victorian Branch.

Walby, S. & Soothill, K. (1994). Medicine and nursing: professions in changing health service. London: Sage Publications.

Wood Report (1947) *Report of the Working Party on the Recruitment and Training of Nurses,* Ministry of Health, Department of Health for Scotland and Ministry of Labour and National Service, HMSO, London.

## RECOMMENDED READING

Braverman, H. (1974). *Labor and Monopoly Capital: The Degradation of Work in the Twentieth Century*. London: Monthly Review Press.

DEST. Department of Education, Science and Training (2002). *National Review of Nursing Education 2002: Our Duty of Care*. Canberra, Australia.

Flanagan, J. (1998). Achieving partnership: The contribution of nursing education to the production of a flexible workforce. *Journal of Nursing Management*, 6, 129–136.

Meadows, G. (2002). The nursing shortage: Can information technology help? *Nursing Economics*, 20(1), 46–48.

# Research and Scholarship for Technology and Nursing

## Alan Barnard

---

When you have read this chapter, you will be able to:

- Discuss the relation between nursing, technology and research

- Identify the importance of research and scholarship for future nursing practice and health care

- Identify research perspectives common to examining technology

- Consider research and scholarship in relation to professional advancement

- Highlight the importance of research and scholarship for person-focused care

---

═══════════ **KEY WORDS** ═══════════

- clinical practice

- evidence

- nursing

- research

- technique

- technology

- scholarship

---

## 11.1 Introduction

Technology is a significant influence on cultural, professional and social development and needs to be examined through appropriate research and scholarship (Ihde, 1993, 1995; Illich, 1976; Pacey, 1983; Reiser, 1978). It has an ability to influence people and health care and we nurses are important to the efficiency and effectiveness of technology. Our roles and responsibilities reflect a history, culture and future linked with technology (Barnard & Cushing, 2001; Fairman, 1998; Sandelowski, 2000). It is not surprising that there is growing interest in highlighting not only 'what we do as nurses' but 'why we do it'. Our contributions to health care and the influence of technology is profound, yet they remain significantly under-acknowledged and under-represented in health care research.

Research and scholarship is needed now that shows the complexity of technology. Brey (2003) and Feenberg (2003) note that in many ways professions such as ours need to engage in both micro and macro analysis of technology using both quantitative and qualitative methodology to focus on the development of a fair and just society. Micro-analysis examines the relations between technology and health care practice(s) as well as change to knowledge and skill(s). Micro-analysis might focus on for example, specific technical practices, specialist skills, management techniques, protocols and equipment development, in addition to professional relations, management of resources and opportunities to skilfully utilise technology in care. Macro-analysis is centred on global issues such as rationality of work, efficiency as a health care goal, health policy, the politics of care, organisational systems, historical and futurist accounts of technology, cultures and society. Even though macro-analysis provides a rich and comprehensive addition to technology research and a different level of analysis and understanding, this area of research is neglected in nursing and health care. The reasons for the neglect are speculative but relate in the first instance to the fact that technology is equated often with technical practice and material purpose rather than in relation to other significant factors in the context of practice and society (Barnard, 2002; Bunge, 2003; Ellul, 1980; Sandelowski, 2000).

Although nursing is informed by science, the practice of nursing is fundamentally a technology. We are engaged often in practice in which our primary interests relate to people and practical results, whether in relation to, for example, wound care, changing health behaviour, accessing information or encouraging persons to express their feelings. We make use of fundamental scientific knowledge related to, for example, mathematics, biology and the humanities to form specific knowledge and skills that are expressed through practical reasoning. We nurses have positioned ourselves importantly yet precariously in the space between technology and human experience. The position is precarious because it is a challenge to ensure we expertly respond to both sides of the boundary. For example, it is stated often that some nurses do not care enough about their patients because they are too busy looking after machinery and, alternatively, that some nurses are disinterested in new technology and fail to adequately learn how to integrate technologies best into practice.

We make a profound contribution to health care and are concerned about both the application of technology and the daily experience of persons. The breadth of research opportunity is enormous. Much like the ways different layers of an artist's painting come together to form a complete picture, our orientation to care ought to be guided by an emphasis on appropriate, safe and competent practice using technology; skills informed by evidence, knowledge and critical thinking; and a philosophy to care that affirms always the importance of human dignity and worth.

Research studies that focus on nursing perspectives in health care are growing and there are a plethora of key professional and social questions associated with, for example, eHealth, genetics, technology assessment, visual representation, information technology, informatics, practitioner skills and knowledge, specialisation, efficiency, technology design, the sanctity of human life, professional boundaries and the freedom of practitioners to express caring in health care delivery. In this chapter we focus on the importance of research and scholarship with specific emphasis on technology.

## 11.2   An invitation to inquiry

Research that explores technology will assist to improve clinical practice and patient care. Walters (1995) highlighted its importance when he stated that 'As nursing is practiced in the midst of technology, acknowledging the material world of health care involves developing an understanding of technology used by nurses in their daily practice'.

A range of qualitative and quantitative methodology and method is appropriate. Our focus should be no different to any other profession since we too seek to complete scientific research to understand how technology contributes to the achievement of desired health care outcomes (Marck, 2000; Ray, 2001; Sandelowski, 2000; Wilkin & Slevin, 2004; Williams & Umberson, 1999). The range of questions that can be posed by you as a researcher are to a large degree dependent on your interpretation of technology. As I outlined in Chapter 1, a limited definition of technology is unsatisfactory because closure occurs to our thinking. There arises a tendency to focus only on the function of equipment etc., in our action and care. Consequently it is easy to overlook for example, topics addressed in this book related to: care environments and ward design; knowledge change and competency; technology design and its influence on skills; caring practices; or the evolution of health specialties and the division of labour. All these issues and many more have enormous implication for the quality of nursing and the way people are treated in health care.

It is argued that a type of thinking is required from you that acknowledges both our ambivalence (Hawthorne & Yurkovich, 1995; Peacock & Nolan, 2000; Sandelowski, 2002) and excitement about technology (Gordon, 1992; Simpson, 2003). There is a need to rise above assumptions about our work and technology that emphasise an incorrect faith or fear of technology development and progress (Barnard, 1997, 1999; Herdman, 2001; Purkis, 1999; Ray, 2001; Sandelowski, 2000). Like the rest of our society, nurses have a tendency to be both intrigued by scientific and technological discovery, yet have a tendency to express both a fear of technology (dystopian) (Calne, 1994; Donley, 1991) or overly eager presumptions about its benefits (utopian) (Salmon, 1969, 1977; Simpson, 2001; Simpson & Brown, 1990). For example, it is commonplace to claim the benefits of technology without due reliance on evidence (e.g. technology saves us time). It is commonplace to be impressed by the promise of future progress and be swept along by media coverage of technological and scientific advances; however, in nursing and health care we need more. We need to be engaged in sophisticated enquiry into technology and especially focus on the ways in which it does or does not assist health care delivery. In order to do this we require informed and critical approaches to research that seek genuine evaluation and advancement of appropriate care.

The influence of technology on our society and personal lives is so dramatic that it is reasonable to ask 'to what extent does technology influence our practice'. Technology has been linked to alienation of people, professional change, increasing opportunity and dehumanisation. Numerous nurses have argued that technology *forces* change to our day, values, practice and professional lives (Allan & Hall, 1988; DeVries, 2000). Further to this, Postman (1992) has noted that medical practitioners are often dissatisfied with the effects of technology on their clinical practice. Technology has been awarded a place in determining and redefining what doctors and nurses do and for changing how professional groups view people and illness.

Responsibility for the future of nursing and health care involves more than just accepting change and learning to use machinery and equipment. We are required now to make decisive and informed decisions about appropriate care that is based on evidence and insight. Well-targeted and designed research will advance evidence, focus skills and promote professional growth. We now have an opportunity to turn towards technology in order to examine how we can further facilitate meaningful and worthwhile health care practices. As researchers we have the potential to make a profound contribution to nursing, health care and society(ies).

## 11.3   Perspectives that inform technology research

Given the breadth of possible research questions, it is worthwhile considering general approaches to thinking about technology research that inform the types of research projects that might be initiated. If our current and future research follows trends in other disciplines there is likely to emerge a tendency towards either social constructivist or substantivist perspectives.

### The social constructivist perspective

Social constructivism focuses on social alliances that are important to technical choice. Social constructivists explore how social alliance (networks or collaboration between people and groups) determine the outcomes and development of technology. Technology is interpreted as a servant of values and goals.

For example, changes to your clinical practice and the workplace are argued to reflect factors such as 'the way we get along' and the subsequent design of technology rather than any pre-determined scientific-technical logical order belonging to technology. Research questions that emerge from this perspective focus primarily on the knowledge, legitimacy and relationships between the various people (actors) involved in the use, design and integration of technology. Social alliance and interest can foster or impede technology (Feenberg, 1999) and there are examples of nurses who share this view. Published research has focused on, for example, the integration of computers in health care, the development of a telehealth facility for psychiatry in the community, and strategies to reduce nurse 'resistance' to the better use of information technology in clinical practice (Alexander & Kroposki, 2001b; Hepworth & Fitter, 1981; May, et al., 2001; Wilkin & Slevin, 2004).

The primary focus of social constructivist orientated research is on the knowledge and legitimacy of all the various actors (e.g. nurses) involved in the use and integration of technology. The principal aim is to identify how technology operates in relation to human affairs. Variation in human experience as it relates to the experience of technology is acknowledged yet minimised since technology and the world 'lived' are understood from a mechanistic or functional viewpoint. Successful social and professional change is attributed to relations between people and groups who are responsible, for example, for the use of machinery, technology design and the management of systems.

The perspective is criticised by Brey (2003) and Winner (2003) as a modern form of idealism which unrealistically ignores the fact that technology is a phenomenon that has a determining influence on society, groups and individuals. A principle criticism of social constructivism is the tendency towards a dualistic approach to research. That is, the perspective tends to split issues and concepts into two separate halves. For example, a renal dialysis machine would be a technological device separate, at least conceptually, to the values and experiences of the person to whom it is attached. Research projects reflect an ontological separation between technology, individuals, groups and/or society(ies) and have a tendency to create disconnection or boundaries between, for example, things that are technical and personal experience; things that are technical – the meaning or values or people; and things that are technical – normal cultural and social practice(s) (Feenberg, 1999). In addition, serious consideration of ethical and political dimensions of technology are sporadic and the perspective encourages us to become therefore, somewhat reactive rather than proactive when confronted by issues related to human values, professions and culture (DeVries, 2000; Herdman, 2001; Marck, 2000; Rogers, Karlsen & Addington-Hall, 1999).

### The substantivist perspective

Substantivist research seeks to examine technology in relation to both what we do and how the world is both experienced and altered by technology. The research perspective acknowledges the importance of the agent or person(s) involved with technology but research questions stress technology as a phenomenon not subject always to the outcomes of social alliance, networks or design. Technology is interpreted as more than machines, good design, skilled management and a collaborative social network. Research questions and methodological assumptions focus on the view that living with technology is more than the good use of appropriately designed technology within strong actor-networks (Feenberg, 1999; Mitcham, 1994).

Substantivist research tends to pose questions that presume technology is always to some extent a determining factor in all our activity and relations. Technology is argued to be a phenomenon that has a bias towards rational control and efficiency, sometimes at the expense of human interests. Design of technology brings with it gendered, cultural and political values and always a potential for unpredicted outcomes. Technology transforms many of our actions, goals, culture and values in search of greater efficiency and control. Research projects seek to show how technology works directly to change nursing prac-tice and health care delivery. Research questions might focus on, for example, the relations between technology and caring in intensive care, freedom of choice and therapeutic relations in clinical practice. For example, Barnard (2000) demonstrated that technology influences nursing practice despite prior experi-ence, social alliance, skills development, knowledge and a desire to practise in a caring and person focused manner. Research found that technology to a greater or lesser extent can influence a nurse's freedom to determine individual goals, care and practice principles. Nursing practice was altered by the demands of technology(ies) which commanded significant attention, time and commitment from nurses.

The perspective is useful for nursing and health care research but it is essential to be aware of limitations. Criticism of substantivism can include unrealistic and sometimes excessive arguments in favour of technological determinism. That is, they argue that technology (in varying degrees depending on the author) will determine actions, people, values and events. There is sometimes also a lack of emphasis on how technology design can influence the success of technology, and a tendency to encourage thinking that builds on a fear of technology and places people in opposition to it (Feenberg, 1999, 2003).

## Developing new research

Although there are challenges, social constructivist and substantivist perspectives offer important insights for furthering health care research and offer a start to what is lacking often in current research, that is, coherent frameworks for interpreting technology, nursing and health care. We need to interpret care using frameworks broader than, for example, an economic perspective that seeks merely to ask 'how much does it cost' or instrumentalist frameworks that merely 'measure activity and action'. Knowing the answer to incorrect or poorly considered questions does not benefit health care, evidence accumulation or scholarship. You might ask 'what is a *new* research about technology' because 'don't we do research already'?

Researchers do examine technology but a significant proportion of published nursing research lacks critical analysis informed by theoretical frameworks to assist interpretation. It is commonplace to ask functional or 'doing' research questions such as 'what is the best way(s) to wean a patient from a ventilator', or 'which hand wash is best for improving cleanliness', or 'how can we get nurses to use (integrate) computers better in their practice'? These questions are extremely important but in no way reflect the scope of potential research areas in nursing and health care. A new approach to researching technology and health care will not be looking 'backward' in relation to problems or possibilities, but will be forward oriented in seeing challenges before they worsen and seeking to identify areas for future development. There will be a focus on the things themselves, but in addition we will be required to ask in what ways specific technologies enhance quality of life and play a positive role in the day to day culture and experience of people. The focus for future research has to be on the appropriateness of technology within contexts and the ways artefacts, systems and resources do, or do not, meet the needs of people, groups and societies. We need less techno-phobia and less techno-utopianism and more targeted and critical examination of benefits and failings.

## 11.4  Research about technology and nursing

Technology introduces patterns of activity and thinking that by their very nature change nursing and lead always to a range of positive and negative outcomes for people and health care (Barnard & Sandelowski, 2001). Thalidomide was good for nausea during pregnancy but caused deformity in the new born. Electronic sphygmomanometers make blood pressure monitoring efficient but lead to skills change in clinical practice. There are causes and antecedents for every action and equal reaction to arise from our inclusion of technology which demand our attention. Discernment of desired care and preference that meet individual and cultural needs are key features of appropriate care and demand our research and scholarship.

There is a growing pressure to make evidence clear in order to inform practice and advance care. The approaches to interpreting technology advocated in this book highlight that our attention could be on more than just technical things. Foremost research and scholarship acknowledge the artefacts and technical things of health care and places that understanding within the context of the greater emergence and influence of technology. Examples of recent research and scholarship include enhancement and substitution of the body; technology, human relations and care; and the challenge of technique.

### Enhancement and substitution of the body

Technology provides prosthetics for natural and acquired physical impairment and often provides the means for people to reach their goals in life. Technologies such as artificial ventilation for chronic illness at home and robotic assistance for the disabled are examples presented in this book of many emerging developments that have the potential to enhance quality of life for many people. Substitution or enhancement of 'the body' through technology has been achieved through the use and development of, for example, artificial limbs, dentures, pacemakers and reading glasses. Technology can restore body function and can also reduce physical limitation. It can have significant psychological impact on the way we understand our bodies, what is defined as an embodied experience and where does my body begin and end. For example, Barnard & Sinclair (2006) highlighted the significant influence technology can have on both the physical presence of the nurse in a care environment and the changing boundary associated with a patient's body as a result of monitoring and surgical procedures. These experiences underpin questions of human meaning, psychological development, nursing theory, practice goals and issues related to changing personal space and social relations.

Technology is incorporated increasingly *into* and *with* the body. The body has become a site for alteration and manipulation. For example, cosmetic surgery and artificial implants to lips and breasts reflect Western social norms associated with beauty, body size, gender, aging and fitness. We have gained the ability to 'shed our skins' (Stelarc, 1998) as our body adapts to cope with the pace of life and our awareness of who we are as persons. However, changes to the human body as a result of technology alter conceptions of being human. For example, cyborg development has implication for gender relations and understanding the human body (Haraway, 1995); cyborg meaning a hybrid of organism (person) and machine (technology) that represents a clear alteration of the boundaries between human and technology and a fusion of nature and culture – a cyborg is a person whose physiological functioning is aided by, or dependent on, a mechanical or electronic device such as an artificial heart, permanent ventilation or artificial hip. Associated concepts and issues related to being human are important for health care and nursing and we are positioned to lead research and scholarship.

## Technology, human relations and care

The 'bed' has historically been a nursing focus and is the quintessential technology of nursing. It is a major point of human interaction, gathering, human care, peace and suffering. It is the definitive technology of nursing. For example, nurse practitioners gather around the bed to 'hand over care', provide care for people, listen to the patient and learn to nurse. It is a focal point that can reasonably be labelled a 'nursing space' but its context is changing rapidly. For example, there are changes to health care provision and environments of care, with particular reference to a growing emphasis on visual representation through eHealth. Electronic and computerised technology emphasise a reliance on quantitative evidence that is available via digital display, computer screens and printouts. There is increasing alteration to traditional relations between nurses and people. The point of care is changing as a result of the development of ambulatory monitoring and tele-health. Technology continues to be a mediator between people and has now created a physical distance between the health care provider and the patient. Changes highlighted in this book attest to these developments and include critical care practice, autonomous and remote presence robotic assistance and home care for people with chronic illness.

Although post-modern thought challenges notions of what is human and natural, nurses are a group among many who still adhere mostly to a humanist view. We have positioned *ourselves* on the *human*/natural side of supposed *human* and non-human and *natural* and artificial divides. We portray ourselves as a bridge spanning a divide between technology (interpreted generally as artefact and machines) and humane health care (that is human-centred and person-focused care) (Cooper, 1994; Gordon, 1992). We have claimed professional ownership of an imaginary space between technology and the patient. Paradoxically, although we occasionally question the influence of technology on nursing practice, we have strategically embraced technology to advance our profession even though we sometimes despise it (Fairman, 1998; Sandelowski, 1999; Walker, 1970). Despite the years of conjecture, what remains unknown is the extent to which technology actually dehumanises, depersonalises persons or actually causes poor care. Research may show that it is not technology per se that causes a lack of caring, but specific user contexts, the meanings attributed to technology, how individual or cultural groups define what is human and an unreasonable emphasis on efficiency and control. It might be better to concede that much of the power of technology is derived from its meaningfulness as a means to influence our actions and thought than its ability to determine care.

Research is needed that explains how technology is best integrated to foster person-focused care. Research might find that the problem of technology lies less with itself than with our understanding, the choices our patients and we make about what is appropriate, natural and dignified. A dignified birth might thus entail a 'low' or 'high' technology presence. Resolution to the problem of 'what is appropriate' is, in part, to ascertain and honour the varied choices and respond to preferences in specific ways.

## The challenge of *Technique*

Our world at one level is a world of things but at another level it is a world that is ordered systematically. Things arranged around us have associated facts, protocols, behaviours and values, which increasingly define our reality, practice and ways of life. There are associated resources that support safe and efficient care, budgets that account for costs, policy that advises on correct behaviour and benchmarks that inform us if our actions are worthy. Several critics of technology have emphasised the importance of understanding and responding to this overarching system (technique) (Ellul, 1964; Feenberg, 1999; Winner, 1977). Technique, not machinery and equipment, increasingly structures our behaviour, lives and culture.

For example, Moore (1998) notes that the outcome of technology development has not been oppression by machines and tools and so forth, but submission to a kind of machine-ness in our thinking and action. We take account of human, economic and political problems as a matter of policy and planning that determine our future and values, yet paradoxically believe ourselves to be free. Technique does not respond to individual and cultural difference. Its purpose is to reproduce itself; it is the centre of its own attention. When we raise issues of individuality and cultural difference in health care we emphasise the opposite end of technique. It is technique, not technology per se that controls much of our behaviour and attention since we have delegated to systems (technique) the power to determine our decision-making (for example, organisational policy and pre-determined protocols that create sameness in care). We now rely on technique more than we realise, and it is technique that makes contemporary nursing 'technological', not objects, machines, automata or equipment. We are included increasingly in a system (often without due recognition) which requires urgent attention and research since it is technique that often determines our actions, clinical intervention and level of care.

## 11.5 Assumptions to assist future research and scholarship

At the foreground of health care research is the need to improve care, empower patients and develop evidence-based knowledge and skills. The background to these needs must be informed by the following five assumptions which are central to future research:

### Good health care matters because people matter

Health care research and practice must be guided fundamentally by principles and attitudes that promote, establish and protect human dignity. Protection of dignity is central to all that nurses are called to engage in, and is central to the utilisation and integration of technology in care. Good health care matters because people matter and this moral value must be continually emphasised and advanced within health care research.

### Technology is more than machinery and equipment

Technology is more than the sum of things we use. It has characteristic features that include the development of skills, knowledge and the incorporation of social arrangements and values (Feenberg, 1999; Pacey, 1999). There is a lack of research into how technology might be a major determinant in these important areas. The reasons for the lack of acknowledgement in nursing are speculative but include our emphasis on application of technology, our inclination to uncritically embrace new technology sometimes without considering its effect(s) on practice, a de-emphasis on research into the 'dirty work' of nurses in preference for advanced technology and a lack of critical scholarship.

### The right to quality care

Each person has a right to available health care resources and quality nursing. Even though access to technology is sometimes restricted as a result of factors such as physical location and managed care initiatives which place limitation on available resources available within a geographic area, the dignity and worth of each life affirms the view that we are responsible to effectively utilise and integrate appropriate technology.

## Technology research and scholarship is political

Technological changes do not always have outcomes that accord with everyone's interests. For example, there is currently a renewed focus on home care in many countries. The family and carer have in recent years been re-constructed as 'team members' within a multi-disciplinary approach to care (Wang & Barnard 2004). Walters (1995) noted that in health care most technology is controlled and purchased by the medical profession and governed by bureaucratic and administrative power elite. Dominant power relationships control the practice of disciplines such as nursing. Even so, we nurses have typically bypassed technology as a powerful political phenomenon that determines relationships between disciplines and in clinical practice. Funding, ward design, appropriate equipment and resources such as power and gas supply are crucial for excellent care as is, for example, the ability to influence decision making, economic allocation and health care policy. Central to providing care in busy, demanding modern clinical environments is the establishment of protocols and policies that are determined often by external authorities such as health administrators and government departments. The political struggles outlined by Moya Conrick in this book highlight well the achievements that are there to be won through engagement in the politics of technology. Political decisions impact directly on the practice of each nurse, the organisation and patient care (Allan & Hall, 1988; Fairman, 1996; Harding, 1980; McConnell, 1990; Sandelowski, 1988; Walters, 1995).

## 11.6 Technology, research and professional development

Technology is valued as a significant precursor for professional development in nursing and is valued by many as a fix for improving effective service, efficiency, cost cutting, labour force reduction and access to information (Alexander & Kroposki, 2001a, 2001b; Shilling, 2005). Whilst these values are sometimes important, there are other measures of quality care such as human dignity, the sanctity of human life and person-hood. For example, the environmental movement is a potential source to inform research into different ways of thinking about health care (Ferre, 1995; Ihde, 1993). Better use and disposal of health care products and the promotion of healthy lifestyles that are environmentally sensitive and responsive to socio-cultural contexts are a good foundation for health. Ferre (1995) argues that the ecology movement has potential to provide assistance in 'post-modern' (alternative) interpretation(s) of technology and practice. The movement has scope for synthesis of ideas and thinking. It draws on the benefits of modern scientific analysis but is free to establish coherence in thinking which is not bound to the physics-based technological models of the pre and current modern world. There is opportunity for research work that draws on the purposes and values of cultures, people, individuals and groups and emphasises stability, durability, sustainability and satisfaction as dominant considerations rather than maximisation of use, efficiency and rationalism. As is argued by many of the authors in this book, there is scope to interpret nature and the human world as fundamentally inter-twined with the world of techno-science. There are opportunities to make significant contributions to our thinking and our clinical practice that seek to correct what are according to Ferre (1995, p. 131) the two great failures of modern technology 'incoherence, or the failure to achieve synthesis for understanding, and inadequacy, or the failure to include subtle data in the powerful but ideally simplified concepts and models it uses'.

## 11.7 Final reflection

Technology has positive or negative outcomes and will never lead to outcomes that are neutral for all people and groups. Quality health care research requires ongoing critical examination and serious reflection on emerging issues and interventions. We can no longer remain inadequately informed by the false assumption that technology has no effect upon people, context, values and behaviour (Marck, 2000; May, et al., 2001; Sandelowski, 2000). The future of nursing needs to be informed by explanation of technology that reflects accurately both our practice and experience. More research is needed about technology and its relationship to clinical practice, models of care, skills and knowledge development, and a plethora of issues associated with, for example, the meaning of quality care, appropriate technological intervention in treatment and the importance of responding to human experience. Analysis of technology is required that relies less on generalisations about dehumanisation, alienation or uncritical celebration of progress, than on considered research into specific relations between technology, people, nursing care and health care practice.

Professional advancement with technology is appropriate and advancement includes researching health care intervention and commonplace views. The quantity and extent of ongoing change around us guarantees nothing for us about its quality. We need a healthy and radical ambivalence towards technology. Research and scholarship is emerging at a timely moment and offers opportunity to enrich our insight into questions and challenges related to the nature and scope of health care. There is opportunity for us to make a profound contribution.

Future practice will demand further insight into technology in order to equip us to better engage in determining the direction of health care (Fairman & Lynaugh, 1998; Locsin, 1995, 1998; Walters, 1995). Research at this time needs to focus particularly on the suitability of technology for health care provision; advancing person-focused care; identifying sustainable and effective health care initiatives; and re-invigorating cultural, spiritual, moral and social values important to health care professions. To this end, it was encouraging to note that the U.S.A Institute of Medicine report, 2001, entitled *Crossing the Quality Chasm: A New Health System for the Twenty First Century* emphasised the need for patient-centred and performance-based care that is devised around healing relationships and the provision of health care founded on needs and values. We must make informed decisions in our practice and technology orientated research will enrich our profession and equip us for the future. Through research and scholarship we have an opportunity to foster a broader understanding of technology, to examine and modify technological systems and defend and facilitate meaningful and appropriate care.

## LEARNING ACTIVITIES

1. Write a letter to an imaginary friend outlining an experience that you would like to change when using technology in your nursing practice? Highlight the key reasons for the change and how you would research ways to improve the outcomes of care.

2. In small groups list strategies you use to 'keep up' with knowledge and skills development in the workplace. Report to the whole group your most successful strategy and why it works.

3. As a group write on a board the reasons why research and scholarship that inquire into technology and nursing practice are important. Discuss ways to foster this type of knowledge development in nursing and health care.

## References

Alexander, J. W. & Kroposki, M. (2001a). Using a management perspective to define and measure changes. *Journal of Advanced Nursing, 35*(5), 776–783.

Alexander, J. W. & Kroposki, M. (2001b). Using management perspective to define and measure changes in nursing technology. *Journal of Advanced Nursing, 35*(5), 776–783.

Allan, J. D. & Hall, B. A. (1988). Challenging the focus on technology: a critique of the medical model in a changing health care system. *Advances in Nursing Science, 10*, 22–34.

Barnard, A. (1997). A critical review of the belief the technology is a neutral object and nurses are its master. *Journal of Advanced Nursing, 26*, 126–131.

Barnard, A. (1999). Nursing and the primacy of technological progress. *International Journal of Nursing Studies, 36*, 435–442.

Barnard, A. (2000). Alteration to will as an experience of technology and nursing. *Journal of Advanced Nursing, 31*(5), 1136–1144.

Barnard, A. (2002). Philosophy of technology and nursing. *Nursing Philosophy, 3*, 15–26.

Barnard, A. & Sinclair, M. (2006). Spectators & spectacles: Nurses, midwives and visuality. *Journal of Advanced Nursing, 55*(5), 578–586.

Barnard, A. & Cushing, A. (2001). Technology and historical inquiry in nursing. In R. Locsin (ed.), *Advancing Technology, Caring and Nursing*. Westport, CT: Auburn House, pp. 12–21.

Barnard, A. & Sandelowski, M. (2001). Technology and humane nursing care: (Ir)Reconcilable or invented difference? *Journal of Advanced Nursing, 34*, 367–375.

Brey, P. (2003). Theorizing modernity and technology. In Misa, T. J., Brey, P. & Feenberg, A. (eds), *Modernity and Technology*. Massachusetts, MA: MIT Press, pp. 33–72.

Bunge, M. (2003). Philosophical inputs and outputs of technology. In Scharff, R. C. & Dusek, V. (eds), *Philosophy of Technology: The Technological Condition, an Anthology*. Oxford: Blackwell, pp. 172–181.

Calne, S. (1994). Dehumanisation in intensive care. *Nursing Times, 90*, 31–33.

Cooper, M. C. (1994). Care: Antidote for nurses' love–hate relationship with technology. *American Journal of Critical Care, 3*, 402–403.

DeVries, R. G. (2000). *Midwives Among the Machines: Recreating Midwifery in the Late 20th Century*. [Retrived 14 September 2000] http://www.stolaf.edu/people/devries/docs/midwifery.html.

Donley, R. (1991). Spiritual dimensions of health care: nursing mission. *Nursing & Health Care, 12*, 178–183.

Ellul, J. (1964). *The Technological Society*. New York: Alfred A. Knopf.

Ellul, J. (1980). *The Technological System*. New York: Continuum.

Fairman, J. (1996). Response to tools of the trade: Analysing technology as object in nursing. *Scholarly Inquiry for Nursing Practice: An International Journal, 10*, 17–21.

Fairman, J. (1998). The nurse-technology relationship in the context of the history of technology. *Nursing History Review, 6*, 129–146.

Fairman, J. & Lynaugh, J. (1998). *Critical Care Nursing: A History*. Philadelphia, PA: The University of Pennsylvania Press.

Feenberg, A. (1999). *Questioning Technology*. New York: Routledge.

Feenberg, A. (2003). Modernity theory and technology studies: reflections on bridging the gap. In Misa, T. J., Brey, P. & Feenberg, A. (eds), *Modernity and Technology*. Massachusetts, MA: MIT Press, pp. 73–104.

Ferre, F. (1995). *Philosophy of Technology*. London: The University of Georgia Press.

Gordon, S. (1992). The importance of being nurses. *Technology Review, 95*(7), 42–51.

Haraway, D. (1995). Cyborgs and symbionts: living together in the new world order. In Gray, C. H. (ed.), *Cyborg Handbook*. New York: Routledge, pp. xi–xx.

Harding, S. (1980). Value laden technologies and the politics of nursing. In Spicker, S. F. & Gadow, S. (eds), *Nursing: Images and Ideals*. New York: Springer, pp. 49–75.

Hawthorne, D. L. & Yurkovich, N. J. (1995). Science, technology, caring and the professions: Are they compatible? *Journal of Advanced Nursing, 21*, 1087–1091.

Hepworth, S. & Fitter, M. (1981). *Nurses' Attitudes to Computers in Hospitals* (Memo No. 419, MCR/ESCR). United Kingdom: University of Sheffield.

Herdman, E. (2001). The illusion of progress in nursing. *Nursing Philosophy, 2*, 4–13.

Ihde, D. (1993). *Philosophy of Technology: An Introduction*. Indiana, IN: Indiana University Press.

Ihde, D. (1995). Image technologies and traditional culture. In Feenberg, A. & Hannay, A. (eds), *Technology and the Politics of Knowledge*. Bloomington, IN: Indiana University Press, pp. 147–158.

Illich, I. (1976). *Limits to Medicine*. London: Calder & Boyars.

Locsin, R. (1995). Machine technologies and caring in nursing. *Image: Journal of Nursing Scholarship, 27*, 201–203.

Locsin, R. (1998). Technologic competence as caring in critical care. *Holistic Nursing Practice, 12*, 50–56.

Marck, P. B. (2000). Recovering ethics after 'technics': developing critical text on technology. *Nursing Ethics, 7*, 5–14.

May, C., Gask, L., Atkinson, T., Ellis, N., Mair, F. & Esmail, A. (2001). Resisting and promoting new technologies in clinical practice: The case of telepsychiatry. *Social Science & Medicine, 52,* 1889–1901.

McConnell, E. A. (1990). The impact of machines on the work of critical care nurses. *Critical Care Nursing Quarterly, 12*(4), 45–52.

Mitcham, C. (1994). *Thinking Through Technology: The Path between Engineering and Philosophy.* Chicago: The University of Chicago.

Moore, R. C. (1998). Hegemony, agency, and dialectical tensions in Ellul's technological society. *Journal of Communication, 48*(3), 129–144.

Pacey, A. (1983). *The Culture of Technology.* Massachusetts, MA: MIT Press.

Pacey, A. (1999). *Meaning in Technology.* Cambridge: The MIT Press.

Peacock, J. & Nolan, P. (2000). Care under threat in the modern world. *Journal of Advanced Nursing, 32*(5), 1066–1070.

Postman, N. (1992). *Technology: The Surrender of Culture to Technology.* New York: Alfred A. Knopf.

Purkis, M. E. (1999). Embracing technology: an exploration of the effects of writing nursing. *Nursing Inquiry, 6,* 147–156.

Ray, M. A. (2001). Complex culture and technology: Toward a global caring communitarian ethics of nursing. In R. Locsin (ed.), *Advancing Technology, Caring, and Nursing.* Westport, CT: Auburn House, pp. 41–52.

Reiser, S. J. (1978). *Medicine and the Reign of Technology.* Cambridge: Cambridge University Press.

Rogers, A., Karlsen, S. & Addington-Hall, J. (1999). All the services were excellent. It is when the human element comes in that things go wrong: Dissatisfaction with hospital care in the last year of life. *Journal of Advanced Nursing, 31*(4), 768–774.

Salmon, B. (1969). Nursing in the age of automation. *The New Zealand Nursing Journal, 62*(12), 20–21.

Salmon, B. (1977). Look toward that mountain. *The New Zealand Nursing Journal, 70*(4), 17–21.

Sandelowski, M. (1988). A case of conflicting paradigms: Nursing and reproductive technology. *Advances in Nursing Science, 10*(3), 35–45.

Sandelowski, M. (1999). Venous envy: The post-World War II debate over IV nursing. *Advances in Nursing Science, 22*(1), 52–62.

Sandelowski, M. (2000). *Devices and Desires: Gender, Technology and American Nursing.* Chapel Hill, NC: The University of North Carolina.

Sandelowski, M. (2002). Visible humans, vanishing bodies, and virtual nursing: complications of life, presence, place, and identity. *Advances in Nursing Science, 24*(3), 58–70.

Shilling, C. (2005). *The Body in Culture Technology and Society.* London: Sage Publications.

Simpson, R. (2001). Compassion meets the computer age. *Nursing Management, 32*(1), 13–14.

Simpson, R. (2003). Today's challenges shape tomorrow's technology, part 1. *Nursing Management, 34*(10), 16–19.

Simpson, R. L. & Brown, L. N. (1990). How to survive the next decade. *Nursing Management, 21*(12), 24–25.

Stelarc. (1998). From psycho-body to cybersystems. In Bell, D., & Kennedy, B. (eds), *The Cybercultures Reader.* London: Routledge.

Walker, D. J. (1970). Our challenging world. *Nursing Forum, 9*(4), 328–339.

Walters, A. J. (1995). Technology and the lifeworld of critical care nursing. *Journal of Advanced Nursing, 22,* 338–346.

Wang, K. W. K. & Barnard, A. (2004). Technology-dependent children and their families: A review. *Journal of Advanced Nursing, 45*(1), 36–46.

Wilkin, K. & Slevin, E. (2004). The meaning of caring to nurses: an investigation into the nature of caring work in an intensive care unit. *Journal of Clinical Nursing, 13,* 50–59.

Williams, K. & Umberson, D. (1999). Medical technology and childbirth: experiences of expectant mothers and fathers. *Sex Roles, 41*(3/4), 147–167.

Winner, L. (1977). *Autonomous Technology*. Massachusetts, MA: The MIT Press.

Winner, L. (2003). Social constructivism: Opening the black box and finding it empty. In R. C. D. Scharff, V. (ed.), *Philosophy of Technology: The Technological Condition, an Anthology*. Oxford: Blackwell, pp. 233–244.

## RECOMMENDED READING

Sandelowski, M. (1997). (Ir) Reconcilable differences? The debate concerning nursing and technology. *Image: Journal of Nursing Scholarship, 29*(2), 169–174.

# Technological Caring as a Dynamic of Complexity in Nursing Practice

## Marilyn Ray

When you have read this chapter, you will be able to:

- Describe the meaning of technological caring in nursing

- Explain key issues and concepts significant to understanding technological caring and nursing

- Identify the importance of technology in relation to research, future theoretical development and clinical nursing practice

- Discuss technological caring as a dynamic of complexity in the practice of nursing

## KEY WORDS

- caring

- co-creative emergence

- complex organisations

- complexity nursing

- complexity sciences

■ ethics

■ faith

■ hope

■ love

■ presencing

■ technology

■ technological caring

■ trust

## 12.1  Introduction

Technology is a creative, aesthetic and spiritual phenomenon, advanced through awareness of one's situatedness and understanding of one's place in the world. A person is not merely an instrument; therefore, technology is not merely tools or instrumentation (Marcel in Wall, 1977). Technology has a relational identity. Technology is advanced for purposes of human survival, transmission of cultural values, development of societies, economic gain, political leadership, military power, maintenance of health, the giving and receiving of information and exploration. From an anthropological viewpoint, technology emerged in relation to developing tools for survival, and personal and social well-being. Throughout history many philosophers asserted that, through technology, humans can gain mastery over nature, the means to satisfy basic human needs (Bernstein, 1971). The theologian, St. Thomas Aquinas, however, '... viewed the substantial unity of man as the cause whereby matter is raised to a spiritual existence' (Pegis, 1945), that is, all matter is eventually apprehended and directed towards what is truly good and beautiful. Heidegger (1977), a noted twentieth century philosopher of technology stated that in early Greek times, the bringing forth of truth was considered techne, the bringing forth of the true and the beautiful. Moreover, Heidegger saw technology as a means to an end and claimed that the ultimate essence of technology is not only the human beings' concern for uses, products and so forth but the 'coming to presence', the creative emergence of art and truth, ultimately mystery (what is constantly being revealed or unconcealed). Today, technology is viewed generally in terms of two perspectives – social constructivism (social relations that shape technology) and substantivist (technology that shapes society). Science and technology also may be considered as two distinct bodies of knowledge, but in some circles they are considered aligned (Chapter 1). Rather than separateness or alignment of science and technology, often reports show that there is a priority for technology over science (Ihde, 1983). The new sciences of complexity, emerging over the past century, illuminate dynamic interconnectedness, knowledge of technology existing in relationship rather than in the objective world or in subjective experience.

Science is not subordinate to technology; it resonates with it. Through technological advances, complexity sciences illuminate the ontology of holism (unity or order) and the notion of chaos – the whole, self-organisation or order that emerges from disorder at the edge of chaos in complex systems (Briggs & Peat, 1989; Peat, 2003; Ray, 1998a). Winner (1990) argued that contemporary developments in electronics and telecommunication suggest that one could exist in a physical or embodied state but can be disembodied within cyberspace. But the tenets of the sciences of complexity challenge the idea of disembodiment. Everything now is viewed as connected; everyone engaged technologically is enmeshed in the information of his or her own question, problem or, in the Heideggerian sense, the mystery being revealed. Are there keys to grasping the complex nature of the meaning of technology and caring in nursing practice? This chapter will attempt to address challenges facing nursing. First, the central precepts of the sciences of complexity will be offered followed by discourse on the meaning of the personal and the professional in nursing, technology as a relational phenomenon captured as 'the past kept in things' (memory), the 'presence-at-hand' or the meaning of being present with technology, and finally illumination of technological caring in nursing practice exemplar as co-creative emergence portraying both embodiment, the onto-theological and the ethics of trust (faith, hope and love).

## 12.2 Complexity sciences and nursing

Scholars in nursing provide various critiques and theories of the meaning of technology and nursing highlighting the complexity of thinking and understanding (Locsin, 2001, 2005). Technology, touch and the virtual have been highlighted in professional relationships (Gadow, 1984; Sandelowski, 2002). Barnard (2005) claimed that there is no unique trait that characterises an essence that is technology but offers recommendations that nurses can reflect upon and study to improve care through the notion of the right use of technology in nursing practice. As an example, Ray advanced the Theory of Bureaucratic Caring (Ray, 1981, 1989, 2001a) from research on caring in the complex system of the hospital. Technology and caring were determined as interconnected. In subsequent phenomenological studies of caring in critical care units, the underlying ethical and moral process of the nurse–patient relationship of technological caring was discovered (Ray, 1987, 1998b). Another example of technology and caring was advanced by Locsin (1995, 2005). After conducting research, Locsin articulated a model for nursing practice where caring and technology, although interconnected, exist independently of each other; however, technical competency itself is viewed as caring. Despite the hidden nature of the philosophy, research and practice of nursing in general scientific and technological discourse, the complexity of the relationship between human caring and technology makes nursing one of the most complex of the relational disciplines.

### Complexity sciences

Complexity sciences are scientific dynamical theories that illuminate the interconnectedness of all things in the universe. Bohm theorised that the universe was fundamentally indivisible, a flowing wholeness in which the observer cannot be separated from that which is observed (Goodwin, 2003; Peat, 2003). Theories of complexity sciences articulate philosophies and integrate concepts that represent an interrelationship among contemplation (intuition), reason and action. There are 31 definitions of complexity that have been proposed. Common definitions are emergence, belongingness, interconnectedness, network of relationships, chaos (order and disorder), patterning and self-organised criticality (Horgan, 1995). Main subsets of complexity have a bearing on the nature of the universe and technological knowing. Holonomy, quantum mechanics, chaos theory and information theory are subsets of complexity sciences. All theories are integral to the technology that facilitated their evolution. The new sciences have had over a century long journey. The journey is both controversial and volatile but overall, new paradigm thought into nature's wholeness have given shape to the fascinating developments in the philosophy of holism, the sciences of physics, astronomy, communication/information processing, technology, ecology, and a new context for theology, a sense of belonging which is at the heart of spiritual awareness (Capra, Steindl-Rast & Matus, 1991; Rogers, 2003).

Holonomy is the study of the interrelationship between parts and whole where the properties of the parts (explicate order) can only be understood from the dynamics of the whole (implicate order). Holism also relates to ecology which looks at living and non-living things as wholes in the universe but also how wholes are embedded in larger wholes to arrive at the highest common bond of the universe and humanity (Capra, Steindl-Rast & Matus, 1991; Goodwin, 2003).

The traditional science of Galileo, Kepler, Descartes and Newton, continues to have considerable influence by describing most things in mathematical or mechanical terms (Briggs & Peat, 1989). Ancient cosmological views of the universe illuminated a dynamical process, a tension between chaos and order (ancient Egyptian and Babylonian stories, Chinese myths, and Biblical images) (Briggs & Peat, 1989) but these ideas were subordinated to the precepts of traditional science. The history of science over the last three centuries, especially Newtonian syntheses showed that the programmes of science or physics had almost reached completion in terms of concepts of order, determinism and reversibility. For science, phenomena are orderly when movements could be explained in terms of cause and effect and explained by linear differential equations. However, we see that science did not evolve as originally anticipated. Pluralistic views and paradoxical phenomena of the physical world began to emerge. Through theorising and observing, a number of scientists of the late nineteenth and early-twentieth centuries began to understand the nature of the universe more in relation to nonlinearity, turbulence, irregularity, and unpredictability. Poincare, Planck, Einstein, and others were occupied with exhibiting the differences between the classical Newtonian view of nature and the view from the perspectives of theories of relativity and the quantum. Quantum science (quantum energy) did shepherd amazing things – the laser, the computer chip and knowledge of nuclear energy/warfare that transformed the world (Briggs & Peat, 1989). However, the general nature of nonlinearity was not fully appreciated. The strength of Newton's laws of force and mass, and especially the need for predictability and reduction to cause and effect of systems continued to dominate, and often continues to reign. New scientific experimentation through technology showed that phenomena that may appear antithetical actually coexist such as determinism and uncertainty, reversibility and irreversibility. This new vision of matter, the processes shaping nature, no longer was associated with passivity and mechanism but with spontaneity and dynamic activity. In quantum mechanics, physicists learned that an elementary unit of light can behave differently, like a wave or like a particle, depending on what the experimenter chooses to measure. Ordinarily system communication is the key construct but researchers found 'that if two quanta (particles) are separated by several meters with no mechanism for communication between them, they will nonetheless remain correlated in some mysterious fashion' (Briggs & Peat, 1989, p. 29).

Chaos theory also a subset of complexity holds that order emerges out of chaos. Chaos deals essentially with the notion of order within disorder at the system communication point or phase space (where attractors wait) – the edge of chaos. Scientists map or bring into focus, the system's phase space for position and speed. Chaos theory illustrates that 'life at the edge of chaos' or where turbulent behaviour is exhibited is about the search for properties and understanding that govern disorder. Choices in the phase space are recognised and the hidden unity is revealed (Ray, 1998a). Creative emergence is the central quality of the evolutionary process. 'It is relational order among components that matters more than material composition in living processes, so that emergent qualities predominate over quantities' (Goodwin, 1994, p. xii). The discoveries have had an enormous affect on ideas about the relation between hard and soft sciences or simple systems (classical physics) and complex systems (economics or cultural systems) (Nicolis & Prigogine, 1989). Although nursing is not included in complexity philosophers' views, nursing is a complex system, notably because of its philosophies of unitary human persons, and of caring, ideals which unify and enhance the experiences of individuals involved in decisions about diverse ranges of possibilities of being and being together (advocate, counsellor, friend, colleague, facilitator, technician, manager, informatician, etc.) (Gadow, 1980; Ray, 1989, 1994a, b, 2001a, b; Swinderman, 2005).

Despite the movement towards the participatory nature of science and the identification of complexity sciences as the sciences of quality, Information Theory developed by Shannon in 1948 was conceived to *quantify* the information content in a message (Smith, 1998). This hypothesis gave rise to the theoretical foundation for information coding, encryption and compression and other aspects of information processing. The theory, however, lacked a system of meaning (Horgan, 1995). Smith (1998) argued that computer science grounded in computation, must, like cognitive science, develop a theory of intentionality, one where the meaning can be imputed by the integration of retentions (the past), protentions (the anticipated future), within the present of the constituting consciousness (Husserl, 1970; Purnell, 2003; Reeder, 1984). Merleau-Ponty, (1962, xii) stated that 'the whole universe of science is built upon the world as directly experienced', that is, all knowledge is gained from one's own specific point of view, or from some experience of the world without which the language of science would be meaningless. McDermott (1990) reinforced the participatory nature of technology by arguing that things provide us with our most distinctive, albeit failing grasp on our distinctive human project, to survive 'being-in-the-world' (p. 290). Connected practices are the constitutive phenomena of intentionality. Computation, artificial intelligence and cognitive science are viewed as social, as fundamentally participatory and irreductionist (Smith, 1998). Over the past century, the evolution of complexity sciences have presented opportunities for the search for relational order, a unified theory of life – unified patterns within complex, chaotic systems from computer science, astrophysics, physics, biology, genetics, socio-cultural systems including organisations, to human caring relationships. Conversely, perplexity has surfaced with questions about whether or not the possibility that a single unity, oneness or wholeness theory of the nature of the universe and the human's place actually can be achieved (Horgan, 1995).

## Complexity in nursing

From a nursing perspective, Rogers (1970) was the first to integrate the notion of complexity followed by Newman (1986) and Davidson (Davidson & Ray, 1991). Rogers introduced nursing to her theory of unitary human persons, human-environment integrality, pattern recognition, multidimensionality and increasing complexity. Newman advanced ideas for the practice of nursing about health as expanded consciousness. Studying technological environments, Davidson built upon Rogers' theory and used complexity sciences to discover *choice* as the key insight in understanding self and life patterning in the integrality of the human-environment relationship (Davidson & Ray, 1991). The interrelationship between contemplation, meaning and action as choice-making was articulated in the development of complex caring dynamics for nursing inquiry by Ray (1994b) followed by the theory of Relational Caring Complexity (relational self-organisation through ethical choice-making) from research studies of economic caring in organisational cultures (Ray, Turkel & Marino, 2002; Turkel & Ray, 2000, 2001). In the complex economic and technological nursing environment of today, research demonstrates that the nurse co-creates order from disorder (at the edge of chaos) through participatory *ethical* choice-making to facilitate transformation or self-organisation (Ray, Turkel & Marino, 2002). The quest for a unified or standardised communication system is beginning to challenge the relational caring ordering/processing of nursing. By means of a focus on the meaning of evidence-based practice (Mitchell, 1999; Swinderman, 2005; Turkel, in press) as a human science, nurses, especially nurse informaticians, are attempting to come up with content and maps that facilitate the emergence of communication systems for best practices that are participatory, ethical and nurse caring-centred, a philosophy of presence.

## 12.3 Philosophy of presence for electronic communication in nursing

The ethical approach to the integration between computer science/electronic information and the person-in-relationship emphasises the need for a deeper understanding of the philosophy of presence (Smith, 1998; Zerwekh, 1997). Can caring presence represent both embodiment and disembodiment at the same time? An answer can be found in a notion in the sciences of complexity: Creative emergence. Creative emergence is the central quality of the evolutionary process (Goodwin, 1994, 2003). Thus, caring must be integrated within the sphere of technology as a process of co-creative emergence. Swinderman claimed that nurse informaticians actually are engaged in an emerging process; they '... have the ability to act like magnets or attractors and pull transformations in a desired direction' (2005, p. 114). Nurses have the relational power to humanise technology in organisational life. Human and technological patterns can be co-directed within emerging systems of meaning. The philosophies illuminated by contemporary nursing theorists – Rogers, Parse, Newman, Watson, Leininger, Ray, Davidson (Ray, 1998a), Turkel and Ray (2000, 2001) and Swinderman (2005) have shown that nursing is the science and art of co-creative emergence. Co-creative emergence, the science and art of qualities in nursing, reveal the unfolding of the relational caring experience of the human-environment integrality, the goodness, truth and beauty within techno-organisational cultures. Ultimately, nursing research shows that in complex health care environments, the philosophy of holism prevails; there are no parts as such, but a unified whole, a pattern in an inseparable web of relationships.

## 12.4 Technology as the past-kept-in-things and the presence-at-hand

Contemporary nursing as co-creative emergence is reinforced by the idea of receptive presence as the foundation for the nursing practice of presencing (Zerwekh, 1997). Presence has had a long history in nursing and is a dominant concept in the philosophy of the personal and professional nursing inter-relationship (Ray, 1981b; Sandelowski, 2002; Zerwekh, 1997) including the way in which the socio-cultural context as presence plays a role in nursing knowledge, understanding and action (Ray, 1981a, 1987, 2001a). Marcel stated that presence was love (compassion) itself (Wall, 1977). The techno-organisational context resonates with the presencing of the nurse with the patient. Both support the unfolding of significance. Meaning is attributed to technology by knowledge of the 'past kept in things' (technological memory) and the 'presence-at-hand' (relational technology) (Heidegger, 1977). In nursing, communion with the other, and human and technological communication form the foundation for caring in complex organisations.

Buber (in Zerwekh, 1997) stated that '[h]e who calls forth the helping word in himself, experiences the word. ...' (p. 261). Thus, whatever is programmed (the memory of the past-kept-in-things) or programmable within a technology to facilitate helping will, in turn, help the person who is 'coming to presence' with it. These notions afford a deeper understanding of the personal and professional and the intricacy of the technological caring relationship in the nursing situation. Nurses do not just treat the technology as an objective entity but as an object of experience. Nurses actually assimilate technology into the whole, thus the whole in nursing is not only the integration of mind, body, spirit, but also the ethical interaction with the organisation – the technological, the political, the economic and the legal – the interplay between caring and the organisational context (Ray, 1981a, 1989, 2001a).

How does the memory held in a technological context 'enframe' the presence-at-hand to disclose or unfold (Heidegger, 1977)? Technology throughout history has been articulated as efficiency or the structure of thinking leading to efficiency; that is, technology has been viewed as theories of action. When pre-scientific crafts were replaced or explained by rules, technological theories were founded. Technological theories or a system of rules prescribed the course of practical action (Mitcham & Mackey, 1972). In the modern era, technology is considered computational *and* intentional (Smith, 1998). Modern technology exhibits life-centredness (Mitcham & Mackey, 1972). Heidegger's (1977) notions help us to understand technology – the human being's active relation to the world is defined by the concept of concern; concern is the human's relation to things that take on such forms as using, handling, producing and so on. Technology is a type of disclosing of immanent being; it is an energy that is stored up and transformed to serve the needs of human beings. Heidegger claimed that this energy, stored up in the technology, is the attitude of Ge-stell or 'enframing', the attitude towards the world which is 'a way of revealing, having the character of destining [or unconcealment or the coming to presence], namely, the way that challenges forth' (Heidegger, 1977, p. 29). In this sense, the essence of technology is a memory that endures and reveals; it is a humanising experience; it points to the mystery of all revealing – what Heidegger thought of as truth. Getting past the instrumentalism of technology reveals that the essence of technology as coming to presence, the coming to presence of truth (Heidegger, 1977). Heidegger noted that this realm or truth of technology was art, what shines forth most purely or the idea of the beautiful (Heidegger, 1977). 'Computer scientists [nurses] wrestle not just with notions of computation itself, but with deeper questions of how to understand the ontology of the worlds in which their systems are embedded' (Smith, 1998, p. 42).

Smith (1998) reinforced the idea of intentionality of computation and because computational systems are intentional, they represent some aspects of the notion of art or truth that Heidegger spoke of; they represent not just the ontology of computation but ontology of the nature of 'Being' itself. The ontology of intentional consciousness, grounded in human reflection, is the integration of all our retentions (past), all our protentions (anticipations) that come-to-presence in the 'now' of constituting consciousness (Reeder, 1984). This communion between the technology and the person, between the past, the anticipation of the future and the presence-at-hand reveal the interconnectedness. Nurse informaticians, for example, are committed not only to the internal structures of numbers and sequences of the technology and the object-orientation of the computer, but also to the sense-making, the meaning and the mode of presentation of the technology itself that illuminates the value of the nurse–patient relationship, the caring relationship. In a critical care situation, the nurse is not only committed to the way in which the technology as a structure or 'thing' will help the patient but also to understanding how the patient is, in reality, helped by the technology itself. In an online nursing educational course, the nurse is committed not only to how the technology will reveal the informational content to the student but also to the quality of the educator-student nurse, teaching–learning interaction. The implicate–explicate boundary, the whole and the part, of the interrelationship is communicated as a unified whole. Co-creative emergence is continual. This dynamism of techno-organisational caring is embedded in the consciousness of the caring relationship. Computational systems cannot 'think' in advance of everything that will ever be important or is needed (Smith, 1998) but in the dynamics of reflective, intuitive ethical and spiritual knowing through the nurse–patient caring relationship and the enframing of technology, unique and valid insights into decisions and meaning for the patient and nurse are made known. The presence of compassion or 'suffering with' the patient, even if the patient, who is unable to cognitively respond, engenders feelings of communion and love through touch and tone. The mystical presence-at-hand is experienced. The pattern that connects facilitates a knowing that involves a reality greater than selves, a love; I belong to the other as the other belongs to me. Moral blindness (Gadow in Ray, 1998b) or technological objectivity may prevail in some interactions; however, overall in nursing, there is the assumption that a responsible nurse does share compassionately in the life of the other, the patient, so that the good of the patient is honoured. The nurse and the patient are purposeful: the patient as a unique human being in terms of his or her needs and the nurse as unique in terms of his or her professional responsibilities. The co-creativity of emergence of the meaning of the relational choice-making defines their purposes. For both the patient and the nurse in their unique purposes, the interrelationship, the interaction reveals the coming-to-presence of the science of quality, and the art or truth of caring. The 'response is testimony to the love received' (Marcel in Wall, 1977); it is in the realm of the theological and the beautiful (Ray, 1994b, 1997).

## 12.5 The personal and the professional in nursing

Understanding the realm of the synthesis of the co-creativity of the theological and the beautiful requires a clarification of the personal and the professional in nursing in complex technological environments. Gadow's and Ray's philosophies will be articulated. The nurse-philosopher, Gadow, provided an understanding of distinctions between the personal and professional as a philosophy of the ideal. Gadow (1980) claimed that nursing ought to be defined in philosophical terms rather than sociological, that is, in terms of the ideal nature of nursing rather than the behavioural or cultural. Gadow stated that, nursing as a philosophy of care, provides the foundation to distinguish between the personal and professional. A philosophy is an ideal and a behaviour articulates functions. Watson (1985) helps us to understand the ideal in caring. She claims that it is the protection, enhancement and preservation of a person's humanity which helps to restore inner harmony of mind, body and spirit, and potential healing (health). Ray's discovery of caring in organisations shows that caring is understood in contemporary practice as both an ideal and a sociology or culture. Caring is the integration of different expressions of caring that take on the nature of the complexity of humanity, such as the physical, spiritual and ethical as well as complex organisational cultures illuminating the interrelationship among caring and technology, economics, politics and legal dimensions. The syntheses of the dialectical dimensions then are technological caring, economic caring, political caring and spiritual-ethical caring and so forth (Ray, 1981a, 1987, Ray, Turkel & marino, 2002; Turkel & Ray, 2000, 2001). Universally, caring as relational absorbs the meaning of complexity. Caring unifies and enhances the experience of individuals in complex cultures. An exemplar of technological caring is presented to reveal the meaning of complexity, and technological caring as co-creative emergence for both the nurse and patient. The essence or mode of revealing meaning thus relates to how the context and technology enframe (coming-to-presence) the individual in new ways (Heidegger, 1977). 'What is required in the concrete situation [nursing situation] is the kind of practical insight and knowledge [practical wisdom] whose special merit is its [the] ability to grasp what is demanded [the personal and professional meaning] by the circumstances at hand' (Caputo, 1988, pp. 109–110).

## 12.6 The dynamics of technological caring

Heidegger (1977) stated that the essence of technology is coming to presence by the emergence or un-concealment of the past-kept-in things. The essence of nursing is caring, a co-creative emergent phenomenon in this presentation. Technological caring as emergent co-creativity is caring as coming to presence of the science and art of caring-presencing. Technological caring illuminates compassion and self-transcending love (compassion). Love is the creative gift of one to the other, where one is awakened to the value and meaning of the transcendent nature of being found in human experience (Appleton, 1991; Marcel, in Wall, 1977). By engaging, knowing and 'suffering with' the other, the dynamics of presencing allow for decisions to emerge relating to the personal meaning of the experience of illness, suffering or dying (Gadow, 1980; Ray, 1991). We have seen that social, electronic informational technology is emerging as the norm. We also know that everything is interconnected. While machines as yet are not in the same league in terms of intelligent human beings, is it possible that technology as matter also has a spiritual existence as St. Thomas Aquinas (Pegis, 1945) pointed out. Technology is a participant in the support of the decisions. There is a bond – an ethic of trust that emerges not only with the person but also with the 'personhood' of the technology since it belongs to persons. An ethic of trust prevails. An ethic is historical and speaks to how well people relate lovingly or learn how to dwell with each other so that a good can be achieved

(Caputo, 1988). Nurses relate lovingly and aesthetically to the lived body, mind and spirit of the patient, as both subject and object, as both a holistic being in relationship as well as the technology as an object of experience, an energy that facilitates assessment, planning and evaluation of patient needs. As an example, nurses and physicians use computerised robots to represent them to patients and communicate important information to them in operating rooms, hospitals, homes, clinics. What could be viewed as the objective pole or 'what' is intended is now becoming more of a subjective pole, a dynamic act of inter-subjectivity where the person intending is engaged in all the modes of intending that are possible (past, anticipatory and present). The 'what' that is intended cannot only incorporate the act of inter-relational technology but also incorporates the science of 'evidence-based' practice where science, technology and problem solving emerge as a unity that reveals, a oneness with the past-kept-in-things and the presencing-at-hand. The subjective and objective are relational and emerge as the ethic of trust. Patients in these situations experience this interrelatedness as do the professionals. An ethic of trust in the co-creative emergence of presencing in technological caring is essentially faith, hope and love – commitment (faithfulness), compassion (lovingness), conscientiousness (principled), confident (trusting) competent (knowledgeable), communicative (hopeful presencing) (Roach, 2002). Competency in technological caring comes forward by the way in which the trust (faith, hope and love) between the nurse and patient reveal personal and professional meaning.

## 12.7 The ethic of trust in technological caring: An exemplar

Technological caring advanced by Ray (1987, 1998b) in critical care units mirrors Gadow's (1980) and Marcel's (1949, 1951; Wall, 1977) philosophy of the body as a reflection on existence. Subjective existence to find meaning is the goal of our true longings as human beings (Webb, 1988) – seeing, hearing, walking, interpreting, judging, deciding and acting. A technological environment could not exist only as an objective phenomenon because it is not possible for people to lose all their personal identity. Instruments are means of survival and can be seen to form a part of our bodies. It is true with patients on ventilators or pumps or those who have other technological belongings, such as computer-assisted means of communication and so forth. The technologies belong to the body. For the nurse, the technology of the computer belongs to the nurse's body, mind and spirit. For the patient, the technological aide, whatever it may be, belongs to the body, mind and spirit. Technology as caring reveals the 'past kept in things' (the knowledge programmed) and the 'presence-at-hand' (what is being revealed) in and for the presencing in the experience of co-creative emergence, what can be known as the ethics of trust. From a holonomic sense, a person then is a whole where parts become the whole and the whole is embedded in a network of relationships. Intellectual and rational operations are constituted by the subjective process of relating (Webb, 1988). In a technological environment, subjective existence is our actual life, and the object of experience, the technology, is in relationship with it. Both are necessary for survival.

Technological caring becomes an ethical archetype (Ray, 1987, 1998b). The ethics of trust as faith, hope and love are gifts which constitute the presencing between the nurse and the patient (Appleton, 1991). Mapping the dynamic pattern of experience shows that the ethics of trust is the ethics of principle (duty or obligation) and the ethics of caring (compassion as a moral attitude toward goodness) that work together. In the pattern of experience in critical care units, the ethical decisions, moral reasoning and choice-making undergo a process of growth and maturation. When a nurse first encounters a patient whose ventilator is a part of the wholeness of the body for survival, for example, the ethical interaction is a trust relationship, trust (faith, hope and love) in the patient or family member and in the technology. There is a need on the part of the nurses to reach a level of comfort of technical competence, that is, technical competency in the use and application of the meaning of the technology itself and then a level of comfort to not harm the patient or the self by not knowing how to relate to (to use) the technology. After reaching this level of comfort with the technology primarily to do no harm to the patient (non-maleficence in ethical terms and in turn not subject oneself to the potential for malpractice due to lack of knowledge of how to use the technology), there is a shift in valuing. This shift in valuing often comes by virtue of the 'look' of the patient suffering, rather than the science or technology; the value of the 'look' engraves more deeply on the heart than the application of science or technology (Caputo, 1988). Compassion is present but deepens from the 'look'. The face of suffering un-conceals. The presencing of the patient reveals suffering and the presencing draws us into mystery, which is both revealed and concealed at the same time. What meaning does this experience of mystery have for the patient, for the nurse? The body suffering, the body in pain commands respect, the first major ethical principle – respect for person. The philosopher of ethics, Kant, referred to respect as a humbling experience, an experience which inspires awe and fear (Caputo, 1988). Through this awe and fear in the presencing, the nurse grows in human understanding to discern how the technology (in this example, the ventilator) is affecting the patient. The nurse in relationship with the patient, even if unconscious, needs to protect and preserve human dignity. The maturation of love, and moral and ethical reasoning are sharper when decisions relate to the potential aggressiveness of technology chosen for care. When a nurse realises that a patient's suffering is more manifest by the technology, and the patient is not being helped and exhibits more pain, and the situation is increasingly irreversible, a value conflict emerges in the presence with the patient. Heidegger (1977) would call this experience, a danger. The deepening value conflict is motivated by a deepening compassion, a feeling of peril, a feeling of what it is like in the becoming of the other by the 'look' of suffering face to, in essence, 'face' more suffering. When the nurse cares for the other, and is present to the other, there is a conscious interpenetration of the other into the nurse even if there are no words expressed. The nurse can feel the patient's own consciousness. The nurse begins to take a different course of action – make a new decision or choice to protect the patient against the invasion of the aggressive technology itself. 'To respect others is to come under their spell, to feel their influence; it is more like entering a field of energy than meeting up with an empirical object' (Caputo, 1988, p. 275). This field of energy is in a sense an onto-theological experience, a mystery wherein the nurse experiences vulnerability just like the patient, the vulnerability of human existence, the lack of defence against the flow of life or death, the presence of God, or the Absolute, a force so strong that one knows that a loving power is taking the side of suffering (Caputo, 1988); the nurse feels the hand of God and is transformed just as the patient is transformed to a sense of security in the infinite or eternal (Marcel, in Wall, 1977). Caputo (1988) calls this *'the eyes of faith'* (p. 279), where faith is *seeing and feeling the Good,* where one can make his or her way through the pain, to do good for the patient. The meaning is personal and unique for the patient, personal and unique for a family member or significant other but is a sense of both the personal and professional for the nurse. Patients may not be able to make the decision to change a course of treatment but the nurse is obligated to do so. He or she must facilitate this process with physicians and family members. The nurse is motivated towards a new course of action by enacting the principles of beneficence (doing good), autonomy (to allow a choice) and justice (be fair) for the suffering patient. The ethics of trust as faith, hope and love or 'the Good that motivates change' transforms the ethical decision-making process.

## 12.8 Final reflection

Suffering and the ethics of trust and ethical action relate to complexity sciences and co-creativity. The new paradigm of complexity is dynamic, holistic, ecological and transcendental. It captures interconnectedness of all things in the in the idea of belongingness (Capra, Steindl-Rast & Matus, 1991). The technological caring experience as co-creative emergence is a presencing of belongingness. We belong to each other, we belong to the world, and we belong to God or the Absolute through the ethics of trust: faith, hope and love. We are in relationship (Capra, Steindl-Rast & Matus, 1991). Compassion with and for the other engenders a spirituality – communion and mystery where the one who is wounded by the other, becomes the other to facilitate the choice-making at the edge of chaos where self-organising transformation takes place. The patient and the nurse are transformed through ethical and spiritual choices in the relational and mystical caring experience (Ray, 1994b). Nurses are entrusted with the power of belongingness to respond, to act rightly for the good of the other. Heidegger (1977) claimed that the question concerning technology, the revealing and concealing, the question concerning mystery, in the coming to presence, is the coming to presence of truth. Heidegger noted that in early Greek times the bringing forth of truth was considered techne, or the bringing forth of the true into the beautiful. Technological caring is techne. Watson (1985) communicated that health [including a peaceful death] is unity, harmony of body, mind and soul (the idea of the beautiful), and goal of nursing is caring for and helping patients achieve a higher degree of harmony within body, mind and soul which will generate self-knowledge or truth (relational self-organisation (Ray, 1994a)). (Dying and death are types of self-knowledge or truth by enabling the carer to confide the patient to the fullness of the eternal (Marcel, in Wall, 1977).) From the complexity sciences' perspective, self-organisation is order out of chaos. In nursing, self-organisation emerges co-relationally by means of the caring presencing. The relational caring facilitate choices towards transformation of self and other; it is the idea of the beautiful, the truth of the harmony of body, mind and soul. As we question the interrelationship between technology and caring, the more mysterious but the more whole is its essence. In his final analysis, Heidegger (1977) claimed that technology is nothing technological. In nursing, for the nurse and patient, we do know that through the experience of presencing with each other and technology, the co-creative emergence is always revealing a journey of faith, hope and love, the ethics of trust and a way of truth. Technological caring thus is the gift of one to and for the other, the interpenetration of each in each other's lives.

**LEARNING ACTIVITIES**

1. In small groups discuss your individual notions of compassion as they relate to nursing practice and technological caring.

2. Write down ways understanding the paradigm of complexity can assist with health care and nursing.

3. Write a letter to an imaginary friend explaining your strengths and challenges related to understanding suffering and expressing caring in your nursing. When you have finished your letter list and prioritise six ways you will seek to alter your clinical practice to enhance technological caring.

## References

Appleton, C. (1991). *The Gift of Self: The Meaning of the Art of Nursing*. University of Colorado Health Sciences Center, School of Nursing, Denver, CO. Volume 52–12B# 9215314.

Barnard, A. (2005). Understanding technological competence through philosophy of technology and nursing. In R. Locsin (ed.), *Technological Competency in Nursing*. Indianapolis, IN: Sigma Theta Tau, Press.

Bernstein, R. (1971). *Praxis and Action*. Philadelphia, PA: University of Pennsylvania Press.

Briggs, J. & Peat, F. (1989). *Turbulent Mirror*. New York: Harper & Row, Publishers.

Capra, F., Steindl-Rast, D. with Matus, T. (1991). *Belonging to the Universe*. San Francisco, CA: Harper SanFrancisco.

Caputo, J. (1988). *Radical Hermeneutics.* Bloomington, IN: Indiana University Press.

Davidson, A. & Ray, M. (1991). Studying the human-environment phenomenon using the science of complexity. *Advances in Nursing Science, 4*(2), 73–87.

Gadow, S. (1980). Existential advocacy: Philosophical foundation of nursing. In S. Spicer & Gadow, S. (eds), *Nursing: Images and Ideals, Opening Dialogue with the Humanities.* New York: Springer, pp. 79–101.

Gadow, S. (1984). Touch and technology: Two paradigms of patient care. *Journal of Religion and Health, 23*(1), 63–69.

Goodwin, B. (1994). *How the Leopard Changed Its Spots: The Evolution of Complexity.* New York: Simon & Schuster.

Goodwin, B (2003). Patterns of wholeness. *Resurgence, 1*(216), 12–14.

Heidegger, M. (1977). *The Question Concerning Technology and Other Essays.* (Trans. W. Lovitt). New York: Harper & Row, Publishers.

Horgan, J. (1995). From complexity to perplexity. *Scientific American, 6,* 104–109.

Husserl, E. (1970). *The Crisis of European Sciences.* Evanston, IL: Northwestern University Press.

Ihde, D. (1983). *Existential Technics.* Albany, NY: State University of New York Press.

Locsin, R. (1995). Machine technologies and caring in nursing. *Image: The Journal of Nursing Scholarship, 27*(3), 201–203.

Locsin, R. (ed.). (2001). *Advancing Technology and Caring.* Westport, CT: Auburn House.

Locsin, R. (2005). *Technological Competency as Caring in Nursing.* Indianapolis, IN: Sigma Theta Tau Press.

Marcel, G. (1949). *The Philosophy of Existence* (Trans. By M. Harari). New York: Philosophical Library.

Marcel, G. (1951). *The Mystery of Being.* Vol. I–II. London: The Harvill Press Ltd.

Merleau-Ponty. (1962). *The Phenomenology of Perception.* (Trans. C. Smith). London: Routledge & Kegan Paul.

Mc Dermott, J. (1990). The hidden life of technological artifacts. In T. Casey & Embree, L. (eds), *Lifeworld and Technology.* Washington, DC: Center for Advanced Research in Phenomenology & University Press of America, pp. 289–301.

Mitcham, C. & Mackey, R. (1972). *Philosophy and Technology.* New York: The Free Press.

Mitchell, G. (1999). Evidence-based practice: Critique and alternative view. *Nursing Science Quarterly,* 12(1), 30–35.

Newman, M. (1986). *Health as Expanding Consciousness.* St. Louis, MI: CV Mosby.

Nicolis, G. & Prigogine, I. (1989). *Exploring Complexity.* New York: WH Freeman.

Peat, F. (2003). From physics to Pari: Holistic science: A continuing search for answers. *Resurgence, 1*(216), 24–26.

Purnell, M. (2003). *Intentionality in Nursing.* Doctoral Dissertation, University of Miami, School of Nursing, Florida.

Pegis, A. (1945). *Basic Writings of Saint Thomas* (Summa theologiae, I). New York: Random House.

Ray, M. (1981a). *A Study of Caring within An Institutional Culture.* Doctoral dissertation. University of Utah. Dissertation Abstracts International, 1981 (University Microfilms No. 81–27–787).

Ray, M. (1981b). A philosophical analysis of caring in nursing. In M. Leininger (ed.), *Caring: An Essential Human Ingredient.* Thorofare, NJ: Slack.

Ray, M. (1991). Caring inquiry: The esthetic process in the way of compassion. In D. Gaut & Leininger, M. (eds), *Caring: The Compassionate Healer.* New York: National League for Nursing Press, pp. 181–189.

Ray, M. (1987). Technological caring: A new model in critical care. *Dimensions of Critical Care Nursing, 6,* 166–173.

Ray, M. (1989). The theory of bureaucratic caring for nursing practice in the organizational culture. *Nursing Administration Quarterly, 13*(2), 31–43.

Ray, M. (1994a). Transcultural nursing ethics: A framework and model for transcultural ethical analysis. *Journal of Holistic Nursing, 12*(3), 251–264.

Ray, M. (1994b). Complex caring dynamics: A unifying model of nursing inquiry. *Theoretic and Applied Chaos in Nursing, 1*(1), 23–32.

Ray, M. (1997). Illuminating the meaning of caring: Unfolding the sacred art of divine love. In M. Roach (ed.), *Caring from the Heart: The Convergence of Caring and Spirituality*. New York: Paulist Press.

Ray, M. (1998a). Complexity and nursing science. *Nursing Science Quarterly, 11* (3), 91–93.

Ray, M. (1998b). A phenomenologic study of the interface of caring and technology in intermediate care: Toward a reflexive ethics for clinical practice. *Holistic Nursing Practice, 12*(4), 69–77.

Ray, M. (2001a). The theory of bureaucratic caring. In M. Parker (ed.), *Nursing Theories, Nursing Practice*. Philadelphia, PA: FA Davis Company, pp. 421–431.

Ray, M. (2001b). Complex culture and technology: Toward a global caring communitarian ethics of nursing. In R. Locsin (ed.), *Advancing Technology, Caring, and Nursing*. Westport, CT: Auburn House, pp. 41–52.

Ray, M., Turkel, M. & Marino, F. (2002). The transformative process for nursing in workforce redevelopment. *Nursing Administration Quarterly, 26*(2), 1–14.

Reeder, F. (1984). Philosophical issues in the Rogerian science of unitary human beings. *Advances in Nursing Science, 8*(1), 14–23.

Roach, M. (2002). *The Human Act of Caring: A Blueprint for the Health Professions* (Rev. edn.). Ottawa: Canadian Hospital Association Press.

Rogers, M. (1970). *An Introduction to the Theoretical Basis of Nursing*. Philadelphia, PA: FA Davis Company.

Rogers, E. (2003). *Diffusion of Innovations*. (5th edn.). New York: Free Press.

Sandelowski, M. (2002). Visible humans, vanishing bodies, and virtual nursing. *Advances in Nursing Science, 24*(3), 58–70.

Smith, B. (1998). *On the Origin of Objects*. Cambridge, MA: MIT Press.

Swinderman, T. (2005). *The Magnetic Appeal of Nurse Informaticians: Caring Attractor for Emergence*. Doctor of Nursing Science Dissertation, Florida Atlantic University, Boca Raton, Florida.

Turkel, M. & Ray, M. (2000). Relational complexity: A theory of the nurse-patient relationship within an economic context. *Nursing Science Quarterly, 13*, 307–313.

Turkel, M. & Ray, M. (2001). Relational complexity: From grounded theory to instrument development and theoretical testing. *Nursing Science Quarterly, 14*(4), 281–287.

Turkel, M. (In Press). *Creating Caring Practice Environments through Evidence-based Practice*. Marblehead, MA: HCpro.

Wall, B. (1977). *Love and Death in the Philosophy of Gabriel Marcel*. Washington, DC: University Press of America.

Watson, J. (1985). *Nursing: Human science, Human Care*. Norwalk, CT: Appleton-Century-Crofts.

Webb, E. (1988). *Philosophers of Consciousness*. Seattle, WA: University of Washington Press.

Winner, L. (1990). Living in electronic space. In T. Casey & Embree, L. (eds), *Lifeworld and Technology*. Washington, DC: Center for Advanced Research in Phenomenology & University Press of America, pp. 1–16.

Zerwekh, J. (1997). The practice of presencing. *Seminars in Oncology Nursing 13*(4), 260–262.

### RECOMMENDED READING

Barnard, A. (2002). Philosophy of technology and nursing. *Nursing Philosophy.* *3*(1), 15–26.

Locsin, R. (ed.) (2001). *Advancing Technology, Caring and Nursing.* Westport, CT: Auburn House.

Ray, M. (1994). Complex caring dynamics: A unifying model of nursing inquiry.

Ray, M. (1998). Complexity and nursing science. *Nursing Science Quarterly, 11*(3), 91–93. *Theoretic and Applied Chaos in Nursing; 1*(1), 23–32.

# Index